DATE DUE

KEEPING YOUR KIDS OUT OF THE EMERGENCY ROOM

KEEPING YOUR KIDS OUT OF THE EMERGENCY ROOM

A Guide to Childhood Injuries and Illnesses

Christopher M. Johnson, MD

ROWMAN & LITTLEFIELD
Lanham • Boulder • New York • Toronto • Plymouth, UK

Published by Rowman & Littlefield
4501 Forbes Boulevard, Suite 200, Lanham, Maryland 20706
www.rowman.com

10 Thornbury Road, Plymouth PL6 7PP, United Kingdom

British Library Cataloguing in Publication Information Available

Library of Congress Cataloging-in-Publication Data

Johnson, Christopher M.
Keeping your kids out of the emergency room : a guide to childhood injuries and illnesses / Christopher M. Johnson.
pages cm.
Includes index.
ISBN 978-1-4422-2182-6 (cloth : alk. paper) — ISBN 978-1-4422-2183-3 (electronic)
1. Pediatric emergencies—Popular works. 2. Children—Wounds and injuries—Popular works. 3.
Children—Health and hygiene—Popular works. I. Title.
RJ370.J627 2013
618.92'0025—dc23
2013020555

Printed in the United States of America

CONTENTS

ACKNOWLEDGMENTS

I thank my wife, Jennie Crystle, for her idea to write this book in the first place, as well as my able agent, Anne Devlin, for her enthusiasm and guidance. My copyeditor, John Shanabrook, made it the best book it could be. Most important, I thank the thousands of parents who have trusted me to care for their children over the past thirty-plus years.

1

TO GO OR NOT TO GO:
THE PARENTS' DILEMMA

Last year America's 76 million children made 27 million visits to emergency departments. That is around one visit for every three children. Of course some children accounted for more than a single visit. Even so, the fact that a third of all our children are going to the emergency department each year is a sobering statistic. Was your child one of them? If so, you probably know the difficulty in deciding if and when it might be time to take your child there. Sometimes it is easy to know when to make the trip—an obviously serious injury, for example—but often it is very hard indeed to decide. This is especially so for parents of small infants, who account for a large proportion of children visiting the emergency department. Parents appropriately tend to err on the side of prudence; they bring their child in when they are unsure if the problem can wait or not. Usually this means deciding if their child's problem can wait until morning, because three-quarters of children's trips to the emergency department happen during the evening or nighttime.

If you have ever visited an emergency department with your child, you probably noticed that, whether big or small, emergency departments are not set up for efficiency from a parent's perspective. Rather, they are designed to be efficient from both a doctor's perspective and that of a critically ill or severely injured person. They are set up to be ready for anything on a moment's notice. Like a fire department, an emergency department's staffing and equipment arrangements need to be appropriate for a wide variety of worst-case scenarios. Luckily, very, very few of the millions of children who come to the emergency department need these things. But the facility needs to be ready, just in case. This inevitably builds an enormous inefficiency into the system from the overkill of being always prepared for such rare situations.

Many emergency departments also operate walk-in clinics for children, often adjacent to the full department. These too are often cumbersome, inefficient places to get your child needed care. For one thing, since your child's regular doctor is not there, they do not know her. For another, walk-in clinics are expensive to run—not so expensive as a fully equipped emergency department, but still quite costly. Yet another reason to avoid these facilities is this: if your insurance coverage has an out-of-pocket co-pay, as most do, it will probably cost you more than an equivalent visit to a doctor's office. Why is that? The main reason is that although they might have portions of your child's previous medical record to consult, really these new doctors do not know her at all. So they are much more inclined to order tests your regular doctor would not need. Of course if you do not have health insurance, your bill for going to an emergency department or walk-in clinic will be very much higher than it would have been for getting the same care during a visit to a doctor's office.

The fact that emergency departments are structured this way can be an enormous frustration for parents whose child is not critically or even seriously ill. It is just plain hard for parents to know which problems should be seen right away, which can wait for later, and which probably do not need to be seen by a doctor at all. During my years working in the emergency department, I often found that what parents really needed was not so much medical care for their child as simply information; had they already known what I told them during my evaluation of their child, they often could have avoided the emergency department visit altogether, or at least put off their midnight trek until the next day.

This book will give you specific information about the ailments that most commonly lead parents to consider bringing their child to an emergency department or after-hours clinic. The goal is to give you, the parent, insight into how we doctors look at things, how we decide what is serious and what is not. It will also describe for you what care you should expect to receive when you bring your child there, as well as when you should consider insisting on more than is offered to you.

This book is not a substitute for a doctor's evaluation, and it is certainly not an invitation to practice medicine on your children. Nothing can replace what a doctor does. But over the decades I have practiced emergency pediatrics, I have found that nearly all parents, when given specific information about how doctors evaluate children in the emergency department, make excellent decisions about what their child needs. After all, no one knows a child as well as his or her parents.

2

WHAT SHOULD YOU DO?

This chapter will get us started by telling a series of stories—real-life examples I have seen over the years of the illnesses and injuries children get, and for which their parents brought them to the emergency department. At the end of each one I ask this simple, bottom-line question: If this were your child, what would you do? There are various possibilities, ranging from doing nothing to doing the maximum. We will use the following four action plans throughout our discussions.

1. *Watchful waiting.* Observe your child closely to see what happens next.
2. *Call the doctor.* Call your child's doctor, if he has one, which these days often means calling an answering service or help line staffed by nurses.
3. *Go to the emergency department.* Take your child there promptly.
4. *Call 911.* Do not drive your child to the emergency department yourself—call for immediate help.

Each scenario will conclude by telling you the best option to choose. But what you really need to know is the why, the rationale behind the answer. Most of the key components of that rationale are accessible to any parent who wants to learn them. That is the sort of information that will allow you to make good decisions about what is best for your child when she has, for example, a fever and a sore leg in the middle of the night.

This chapter is a gallop through a whole list of things that bring children to the emergency department. It will give you a good idea of where we are headed together. The rest of the book will slow down and use single chapters to examine each item in this chapter's list in detail, explaining what it is, what to look for, and what to do. The chapters will tell you how to approach each situation as we doctors do. These later chapters will use the same scenarios you will soon read about to dig down into the specific things doctors look for. Each chapter will end with a practical checklist of specific items you can use as a guide about what to do.

Our goal is, if possible, to keep your child from even needing the emergency department. If that is not possible, then you should know how best to use this often confusing and frustrating facility to get the appropriate care for your child. The book's last chapter will tell you about that.

FEVER

We begin with one of the most common ailments parents see in their children: fever. A fever can range in importance from a trivial annoyance to a sign of a life-threatening condition. How do doctors decide where in this broad range of possibilities a child's situation falls? Can parents make use of these principles? In fact, we do have some general rules we follow when evaluating a fever. They are generally simple and any parent can put them to good use. For now, though, consider these common examples of children with fever. I will tell you which of the four options you should choose for each scenario, but you will read about the rationale for my advice in chapter 3, which is all about fever.

Watchful Waiting

Your four-year-old son has had a runny nose for a couple of days, but this has not seemed to affect him very much. He is still active and playful, and he is eating normally. Today you notice he coughs occasionally, but he does not seem short of breath or otherwise bothered by the cough. When you are giving him his evening bath you notice he feels a bit warm, so you take his temperature—it is 101.5 degrees. He still seems normal otherwise except for the runny nose and cough. What should you do?

In this case you do not need to do anything in particular, although you could give him an over-the-counter medicine for fever, such as acetaminophen (Tylenol, many others) or ibuprofen (Advil, many others) if he seems to be uncomfortable from the fever. You could consider calling his doctor in the morning if his fever persists.

Call the Doctor

Your eight-year-old daughter is in the third grade. She was well until yesterday, when she came home from school looking a bit droopy and complaining of a headache. She did not eat much for dinner, and afterward she went right to bed, something unusual for her. You cannot sleep much yourself because you are worried about her, so in the middle of the night you go into her room to see how she is doing. She awakens easily and feels warm on her forehead so you take her temperature—it is 103 degrees. You ask how she feels. She replies that she has a mild headache and a sore, scratchy throat. She also has a stomach ache. You turn on the light to get a better look at her. Her cheeks are flushed but otherwise she looks okay. What should you do?

The answer to this one is, for the present, you can give her something for her fever and a drink of something to keep her well hydrated, and both of you can go back to bed. In the morning you should give her doctor a call for advice if she is not back to normal. She may well need to see the doctor, but not tonight. Although some children like this one need treatment, such as tests and maybe an antibiotic, there is no advantage to answering that question to-night.

Go to the Emergency Department

You have a three-week-old daughter. She has been fine since you brought her home from the hospital at two days of age, and she was fine when she saw the doctor last week for a well-baby checkup. This evening you put her down in her crib after a feeding. When you go in to get her several hours later you notice she feels warm to you so you take her temperature—it is 102 degrees. She may be a bit fussier than usual and her nose is a little stuffy, but overall she does not appear to have anything in particular wrong with her—just the fever. What should you do?

The right thing to do in this scenario is to take your child to the emergency department, even if it is during the middle of the night. As you will read in chapter 3 about fevers, the possible causes of an elevated temperature in this age child are potentially much more serious than those we see in an older child. So she needs to be examined by a physician and will need several tests to look for a cause of the fever. The odds are overwhelming she will be fine, but the risk of not having her evaluated is significant. It is not an emergency requiring a 911 call and an ambulance ride, but she should be evaluated promptly, within a couple of hours at most.

Call 911

Your two-year-old son has been cranky with a fever all afternoon. You gave him some acetaminophen (Tylenol, many others) for the fever and it seemed to help. This evening, though, he did not eat anything at all for dinner and seemed more listless. You put him in his crib and then go to check on him a couple of hours later. He feels hot to your touch, so he clearly has a fever again. What bothers you more than his fever is that he does not respond to you at all, even when you pick him up. He is limp as a dishcloth. His complexion is washed out, even grey-appearing. His breathing is very shallow; as you watch him there are moments when you wonder if he is breathing at all. When you shake him a little he only moans. What should you do?

The best thing to do here is to call 911 for help. He is likely very ill. The possibilities of what is wrong with him are many, and he needs to be seen in the emergency department as soon as possible. He may also get worse quickly. The paramedics that a 911 call brings to your house have the tools and the expertise to take care of that possibility.

COUGHS, SNEEZES, SORE THROATS, AND EARACHES

Upper respiratory symptoms—runny nose, sneezing, cough—are a common reason for parents to bring their child to the emergency department. Some days, especially during the winter, they account for a quarter or more of all the children in the waiting room. As a general principle, however, very few of such children need to be seen in the emergency department in the middle of the night. Fewer would be if their parents knew some of the things you will learn in chapter 4. Here are a couple of scenarios that illustrate some of the possibilities. None of them require a 911 call.

Watchful Waiting

Your two-year-old has had a cough and runny nose for a couple of days. It seems to come at random times during the day, although she does not wake up at night coughing. She also is eating well and has her normal level of activity. She has had no fever. The cough is mostly dry, but every now and then it gets wetter and she coughs up some phlegm. It is Friday evening and your family is leaving the next day for a week-long trip out of town. The cough seems worse, although your daughter is otherwise acting the same. You are worried about her getting worse during the trip and that maybe something needs to be done now for her. Does it? Should you give her a dose of an over-the-counter cough medicine?

The answer to this one is unless she gets new symptoms, there is no particular reason for her to see a doctor. There is nothing a doctor will do at this point that would make much difference, no tests or treatments needed. The answer is also no on the cough medicine. The American Academy of Pediatrics, the professional organization of our country's pediatricians, has studied the subject in detail and found that over-the-counter cough remedies do not work and can cause unwanted side effects. (You will read more about this later.)

Call the Doctor

This case also involves a cough, but this time it is in your six-year-old, who has been intermittently coughing for weeks. You have noticed it is worse at night, and particularly worse after he has been running around for a few minutes. This evening he was out playing vigorously with his friends and came back in the house with a coughing fit. The symptoms are much better now, a half-hour later, and he is now playing comfortably without being short of breath or coughing. You wonder if you should get him checked out tonight because, although you realize the cough has been going on for a considerable time, you are concerned his worse episode tonight means he needs to see the doctor now.

In this situation your child does not need to go to the emergency department tonight, but you should call the doctor about his problem within the next day or so. With these symptoms, the doctor will likely want to see him for an evaluation, especially if his symptoms worsen. His particular breathing problem, which you will learn about in chapter 5, would likely benefit from evaluation and treatment. But it is not an emergency, or even urgent; it is just something that needs attention.

Call the Doctor

This time your two-year-old has had a runny nose and cough for a couple of days. Now at midnight his congestion is much worse, and he has a fever of 103 degrees. He is also digging in his left ear as if it hurts. He has had several ear infections in the past and they all started the same way: a couple of days of runny nose, followed by a fever and fussiness that heralded the beginning of the ear problem. You think he probably has another one. He is irritable, but alert. What should you do?

The answer is that if he is still sick in the morning, you should call his doctor for advice. He may indeed have another ear infection because they commonly follow several days of cold symptoms, especially in toddlers who have had ear infections in the past. The important thing to know is that although we used to assume as a matter of course that earlier treatment of an ear infection makes the child get better faster, later research has shown this is not really the case. Some children may not even need treatment. For tonight it is safe and reasonable to give him acetaminophen (Tylenol, many others) or ibuprofen (Motrin, many others) for his fever and ear pain and to give his doctor a call the next day. There would be nothing wrong with bringing him in for an evaluation the next day, but a phone call might save you the trip.

BREATHING TROUBLES

Difficulty breathing is an extremely common reason for parents to bring their child to the emergency department. By breathing troubles I mean things more severe than just coughing, sneezing, and runny nose. Chapter 5 will tell you all about common childhood breathing problems, how we treat them, and when to worry. You will also learn what sort of breathing is normal for a particular child and what is not, because that varies with age and other things. Meanwhile, here are some common examples we see in the emergency department; some need to be there, but some do not.

Watchful Waiting

Your six-month-old child has had a mild cough for several days. He has otherwise been normal in his activity, eating, and sleeping. Now you notice he has a fever of 101 degrees. You know that the fever by itself is not a reason to do anything other than perhaps give him medicine for it. But when you look at him lying on his back, it seems he is breathing faster than normal. You read somewhere that breathing rate is important, and you time it with your watch; he is taking about forty breaths each minute. His breathing is not labored in any way—it just is a bit fast. What should you do?

In this situation you can just watch and see how he does, see what happens next. His breathing rate is a bit faster than is normal for his age, but by itself that does not mean he needs to be seen by a doctor. For one thing, fever increases breathing rate in many children, so just giving him something for his temperature will often bring his breathing rate down. As long as he does not get worse breathing symptoms, and does not develop any of the particular things you will learn about in chapter 5, you can just watch and wait.

Call the Doctor

Your three-year-old daughter has been coughing all day. The cough is dry, without any phlegm, and as the evening progresses it sounds more and more like a barking seal. She is eating and drinking normally and has no fever. In between her coughing spells she is breathing normally. What should you do?

Your daughter has typical croup, an irritation of the upper airway and vocal cords. You will learn all about croup in chapter 5, but for now here are some useful facts. Croup can be a challenge for parents because it can range from a trivial problem to a severe, even life-threatening one. There are some very specific things to look for to help decide how severe it is. For your daughter's situation, a call to the doctor would be very helpful because the doctor can help you assess how severe the situation is. At this point your daughter does not need to go to the emergency department, but that could change.

Go to the Emergency Department

Your six-year-old son has had a chronic cough for months. It is especially worse after energetic playing. It has always passed within an hour at most. Tonight, though, he seems to be having more trouble. After a summer evening of vigorous running around, he has to sit down to catch his breath. Every so often he seems to heave his chest up higher to get a good breath. When you ask him how he feels, he has to pause and take several short breaths before he can finish each sentence in his answer. What should you do with him?

The answer is to take him to the emergency department. For one thing, he could easily get worse. For another, the emergency department can give him several medicines that will dramatically help his breathing and make him feel better quickly. After he gets better, you definitely should take him to see his regular doctor because he probably will need to take some breathing medicines for several months at least, very often longer. He most likely has a variety of asthma, but he could need some tests to help identify the cause of his troubles. Those are things to deal with later. For now, no matter the time, take him in—every emergency department is well versed in what to do to get him better.

Call 911

This scenario casts you forward a year. In the previous scenario you took your son to the emergency department, he received various breathing treatments, and he got better. They sent him home with some prescriptions for these same medicines, and you took him to his doctor the following week. His doctor said he had asthma and that he should continue to take several of the medicines. A few weeks after that the doctor modified his program a bit, changing him to an inhaled medicine he has taken twice each day since. Overall he has done quite well during the past year. He had a few times when he seemed to breathe harder and have a cough, but taking a bit more of one of the inhaled medicines took care of the problem.

Now he suddenly is having much worse troubles. He seemed fine at dinnertime, except maybe for an occasional cough. Now you awaken in the middle of the night to hear him coughing from down the hall. When you go to his room you find him sitting bolt upright in bed. He can barely speak at all, and with each breath his shoulders rise a couple of inches. You give him a breathing treatment with one of the medications, as your doctor has told you to do in situations like this, and he gets a little better. Fifteen minutes later you give another treatment, but he seems about the same. What should you do? It certainly looks as if he needs more and stronger treatments than you can give at home. Should you call somebody, perhaps the nurse help line your doctor's office uses at night?

The correct answer to this scenario is easy, and it does involve the telephone. But the number you should call is 911. Your son is at risk to get rapidly worse, and the paramedics have all the equipment to bring important components of the emergency department directly to him. He needs to go there, but in an ambulance, not in your car.

DIGESTIVE AND ABDOMINAL PROBLEMS

Abdominal pain, vomiting, and diarrhea are very common complaints in children, and any survey of what brings children to the emergency department contains an ample number of these cases. A major reason is that most acute digestive complaints in children are caused by virus infections—the "stomach flu"—and children get a lot of such viral infections compared with adults. Another reason is that, unlike with adults, it is often difficult for a child to explain just what their symptoms are like. Infants, of course, cannot tell you at all what they are feeling. So an examination by a doctor plays a large role in evaluating what is wrong with them. Most abdominal complaints in children resolve on their own. This can present a problem because parents may minimize their child's symptoms, missing the unusual serious situation that is lurking among all the trivial ones. The following scenarios will show you some of the possibilities. We will explore the specific hows and whys in chapter 6.

Watchful Waiting

Your eight-year-old son has been complaining off and on for several days that his stomach hurts. He is otherwise acting normally and has had a good appetite. You have not noticed anything associated with the pain; it seems to come and go more or less randomly. Now it is evening and he is complaining about it again, although he ate his dinner. He does not seem sick in any other way, but you had a cousin whose child once became very sick with appendicitis, and you know that starts with abdominal pain. What should you do? Does he need to see the doctor tonight to make sure he does not have appendicitis?

This one can be managed with watchful waiting, especially once you know the things you will learn in chapter 6 about appendicitis. He has a stomach ache, but he does not have any of the other things we look for as indicators of serious problems.

Call the Doctor

Your three-month-old daughter has been having watery stools every one or two hours for the past day. She has also vomited up her feedings a few times and seems to be feeding less vigorously than usual. She also seems a bit listless. It is now Friday evening and you are concerned she might be getting dehydrated because you have heard that infants can become dehydrated quite fast. You have also heard there is a blood test that can tell if that is happening. You wonder if you should take your daughter to the emergency department in order to get an evaluation, including blood tests. Should you?

In this scenario it would be best to call your doctor for advice. There are a couple of simple questions the doctor will ask you, and your answers will help determine if your child needs to go to the emergency department or not. It is true both that infants can become dehydrated quickly and that we sometimes use blood tests to help us decide how dehydrated a child is. But generally the answers to some simple questions about the specific symptoms the child is having will answer the question. It is unlikely you would need to bring your child to the emergency department at this time, but some advice about what to look for and what to do now would be very helpful. After reading chapter 6, though, you will know these things yourself, and this scenario could easily move from call the doctor to watchful waiting.

Go to the Emergency Department

This time it is a four-week-old baby who is sick. Like the infant in the preceding scenario, he has been vomiting. But what he has spit up has not just been his last feeding; the material he has vomited is thin and greenish-yellow colored. He also vomits between his attempts to feed, even when there is little to nothing in his stomach. When his vomiting started he kept trying to feed, but over the past several hours he has fed progressively less and less. Another difference from the previous scenario is that, compared with the first child, this one became sicker much faster. Twelve hours ago he was fine; now he is listless. His belly also seems a little puffed out and swollen. If this were your baby, what should you do? Should his parents watch and see how he does, maybe with more-frequent and smaller feedings?

The answer to this scenario is quite clear: this child needs to be seen right away in the emergency department. As you will learn in chapter 6 when we discuss this child's particular problem, the symptoms of vomiting, diarrhea, and abdominal pain span a range of disorders from trivial to quite serious. Even so, it is not difficult for any parent to learn about how doctors separate these possibilities into things needing immediate attention and things that can wait. This boy cannot wait.

Go to the Emergency Department

This six-year-old girl was well until yesterday morning, when she complained to her mother of vague belly pain. She went to school, but when she came home she said she felt worse. She tried to eat a little dinner, but she vomited it all up an hour later. Then she went to bed. When her mother went in to check on her, the child felt warm and in fact did have a temperature of 102 degrees. Her pain was worse. It had also changed in quality; at first it was dull and vague, now it was sharper and worse when she moved. By midnight she had not slept at all, still had a fever, and her sharp pain had worsened to the point that it hurt to move at all. The pain was mostly in the lower-right side of her abdomen.

If this were your child, the best thing to do would be to take her to the emergency department, even if it is the middle of the night. The parent has already used a form of watchful waiting through the evening, and the child has gotten worse—the pain is worse, and now there is fever. A telephone call to the doctor would not be much help because what is most important for this child is an examination by a doctor, coupled most likely with a couple of tests.

BUMPS AND CONKS ON THE HEAD

Few children escape childhood without whacking their heads hard on something, often from a fall from things like trees and bicycles. Since every parent knows that inside the head is the brain, these incidents easily bring anxiety, especially if the child is a bit dazed or acts unusually afterward. Many of the children I have seen over the years in the emergency department have parents who have read or heard somewhere about a minor blow to the head leading to a catastrophic outcome. Their fears are not entirely unfounded—such things happen. But we have good ways of deciding when worrying about the possibility of such a result is reasonable and when it is irrational. Below are some examples. Chapter 7 will explain them to you in detail, along with how doctors sort out head injuries. This will include information about the pros and cons, the benefits and the risks, of commonly used head scans—*computed tomography* (CT) and *magnetic resonance imaging* (MRI) scans.

Watchful Waiting

One evening your ten-year-old is running too fast down a long flight of wooden stairs to the basement. He trips, and tumbles head-over-heels down to the bottom, striking his head on the floor. You hear the crash and find him sitting on the floor. He is a little dazed, but he can tell you exactly what happened, although he scoffs at the suggestion he was running too fast. That is, he has full memory of everything immediately before and during his fall. Afterward he complains of a headache for an hour or so, and he has a lump on the back of his head that is a little tender to the touch. You are concerned, but you think he is probably fine. A few minutes later he is completely alert. Should you take him to the emergency department at this point? Does he need any x-rays or scans of his skull and brain?

The answers to these questions are that this child can be safely observed at home and does not need any x-rays at this point. In chapter 7 you will read about exactly what sort of observation I mean, as well as what changes should prompt you to call your doctor or take him to the emergency department.

Call the Doctor

For this scenario, imagine that the boy from the last scenario, complaining about the pain from the bump on his head, sits down to dinner. An hour later, he complains of some nausea and then vomits. He is still alert in every way, but he feels nauseated. He still has a headache, only now he says that more than just the region of the bump hurts; now his pain is more generalized. It is evening and in a couple of hours it will be his bedtime. His memory is fine—he recalls everything about his fall—but now he seems to be having some symptoms we see with concussions. If this were your son, it would cross your mind that he might have some other reason for nausea and vomiting, the flu perhaps, but he seemed fine earlier in the day. You would not be surprised that the bump on his head hurts, but now his headache seems more than that. If you were in this situation, what should you do?

This example shows how medicine does not always fall into neat categories. This child has had a concussion. Most parents have heard about this condition, and it is a word non-physicians toss around all the time. Most of the time we do nothing about a concussion except watch the child closely. So he does not necessarily need to go and see a doctor now. On the other hand, it is a judgment call, one parents need some help in making. So in this situation it is best to call for some advice. If this were your child and you had no one to call, then it would be best to go to the emergency department, if nothing else to get information and guidance.

Go to the Emergency Department

This scenario features an eighteen-month-old child. She is playing on a screen porch about six feet above the ground. She manages to push out the screen at the bottom of the door, and she then falls down six concrete steps, striking her head on the way down. She has some scrapes, but no significant breaks in the skin. She cries immediately after it happens. Her mother finds her just afterward. The child seems groggy and disoriented, unsteady on her feet. Then she vomits. What should the mother do? Should the child be taken to the emergency department? If so, is it safe for her mother to do so herself, or should her mother call an ambulance?

The answer is that this child should be seen by a doctor. It would be appropriate to bring the child to the emergency department by private car, but a medical evaluation is definitely indicated.

Call 911

For this scenario, imagine the same child is in her parents' bedroom on the second floor and she manages to push out the window screen, after which she falls through the window and lands on her head. (By the way, I have seen many cases similar to these scenarios in which a determined toddler pushes out a screen and falls. Screens are not effective barriers!) Fortunately she hits earth and not concrete. As with the scenario above, other than a scrape there is no break in the skin on her head. The child moves around on the ground just after the impact, really more like thrashes about, and does not really wake up and cry for several minutes. What should her mother do in a situation like this?

The answer to this scenario is an easy one—call 911 because this child needs the immediate assessment and transport skills of paramedics. The odds of everything turning out fine in a scenario like this one are actually extremely good because small children are amazingly resilient creatures, but she needs evaluation in the emergency department, and most likely some scans and other tests. It is safest for paramedics to take her there, and not for you to take her in the family car.

SPRAINS, DISLOCATIONS, AND BROKEN BONES

Children bang themselves a lot. A toddler's natural exuberance exceeds his coordination, with the result that he is frequently falling down. Older children climb things—trees, garage roofs, jungle gyms—and occasionally fall off. Bicycles and skateboards hit fences or slip in a patch of sand. Soccer players collide, baseball players twist an ankle sliding into base. In the last section you read about what to do when a child hits her head; now you will read about broken bones and sprains, about what to do with injuries to the rest of the body, about which kinds need prompt attention, and with which ones you can wait to see how things go. Since most of these common injuries can be managed by watchful waiting, I will give you a couple examples of ones you can safely manage that way.

Watchful Waiting

Your twelve-year-old son falls off a tree limb six feet above the ground. He lands on his outstretched right hand. He comes into the house saying his wrist hurts. You have a look at it. It is not swollen and he can move it around just fine. He is right-handed, and he is able to use that hand reasonably well, although he says it hurts. You check on him an hour later and he is using the hand to play a video game. It still aches, he says. At this point should you take him to the emergency department for a wrist x-ray?

The answer is that it is very unlikely to be a fractured wrist. You can safely give him something for pain, such as ibuprofen (Advil, many others) or acetaminophen (Tylenol, many others), and see how he does. If his wrist starts to swell significantly or the pain persists or worsens overnight (things you will learn to look for in chapter 8), you will have not caused him any harm by waiting— you could take him in the next day to have the wrist looked at.

Watchful Waiting

Now imagine the same son of yours is playing basketball. He leaps for a rebound and, rather than landing squarely on his feet, comes down on the outside edge of his foot, with his ankle turned inward. (An inward-turned ankle is an extremely common injury.) He has immediate pain and limps off the court. An hour later he is still limping, but he can bear weight on his leg. Yet another hour later he is still limping around, so you take his sock off and have a look. Compared to his other ankle, the injured one is a bit swollen. There is a little purplish discoloration. Could this be a broken ankle, or is it just a sprain? And what is a sprain, anyway? When doctors use that word, what do they mean by it? Does he need a late evening trip to the emergency department?

The answer is that, as with his hurt wrist, his ankle is very unlikely to have any broken bones. Guided by what you will learn in chapter 8, a parent can safely follow the same plan with this child as for when he hurt his wrist.

Go to the Emergency Department

You are shopping with your two-year-old daughter. She is at that age when riding in the stroller all the time is no longer fun. She wants to walk around. She darts around a rack of merchandise and you grab her right hand to pull her toward you. She cries out and immediately seems to be holding her right arm funny—she holds it straight and stiff against her body, thumb side in. She also refuses to use the arm. What should you do? Should you watch her overnight and see if it gets better? After all, you did not pull that hard. How could anything be broken?

The answer is that this particular injury is unique to toddlers because of how their arms grow. She has a dislocation in her elbow of a sort you will learn more about in chapter 8. It can be fixed using a specific manipulation of her elbow, but that is something best done by a doctor. Your daughter will feel dramatically better after that is taken care of, but until then she will have a lot of pain and will not be able to move her arm normally. Take her to be seen right away.

Call 9 1 1

This vignette is a tale of two baseball players, both running to catch a foul ball. They collide at high speed and both fall to the ground.

One player gets up rubbing his shoulder but can move his arm around fine. The other one cannot get up, or even move much, because the upper part of his left leg is excruciatingly painful and rapidly swelling. What should be done with him?

This one is simple, and virtually all parents would realize the second child may well have a broken leg. He needs to have that attended to right away. Although the answer in this case is easy, chapter 8 will tell you exactly why that is, about how a doctor decides a fracture is possible, probable, or clearly obvious. Somebody needs to call an ambulance for this child because paramedics will know how to transport safely a child with an injury like this.

SKIN INJURIES

Skin injuries are common. One example is a deep cut, what physicians call a *laceration*. They come in all varieties. There are superficial ones that barely go through the top layer of skin. There are deeper ones that go through to the tissues beneath the skin. And there are very deep ones that penetrate to muscles and vital structures such as bones, nerves, and blood vessels. Every parent knows these most severe lacerations need immediate attention. But what about less-severe ones? The short answer is that all lacerations needing closure are best taken care of as soon as possible. Leaving them open for, say, twelve hours not only can make them more difficult to close later, but can also increase the chances of problems, such as infection or a much larger scar.

Most people know lacerations often need "stitches," or what doctors call *sutures*. But what does that mean? Can some lacerations be fixed without them? Parents really do have a role in making decisions about the specifics of how the laceration is repaired— there are choices in some situations. One of these important choices is painkilling medications and sedatives to keep your child comfortable during the procedure. What about animal bites, like from pets? And what about scars? All lacerations form a scar when they heal. What affects this? Can we do anything about it to lessen scarring? You will learn the answers to these questions in chapter 9.

The skin can be injured in other ways. Heat, in the form of flame, hot objects, sunlight, or hot liquids can cause burns. So can various caustic chemicals. The skin can also be frozen, and that can require medical attention too. What should a parent know about those? There are some handy, simple things you can learn to help you decide when a doctor needs to see your child and when you can safely manage things at home.

Watchful Waiting

Your four-year-old is running around with a ballpoint pen in her mouth. She trips, falls, and bangs the inside of her mouth with the pen tip. She cries, and you see blood running out of her mouth. You help her up and rinse her mouth with water to dilute the blood. You then have a look inside with a flashlight. You see a flap of tissue hanging off the inside of her cheek, oozing blood from underneath it. The gouge underneath the tissue flap is perhaps a quarter-inch deep at most. Does she need to go the emergency department for this?

The answer is that cuts inside the mouth are exceptions to the general rule that lacerations penetrating the skin need closure. The inside of the mouth is not really skin (we call it *mucosa*), and it heals extremely fast. Deep lacerations there, or ones that refuse to stop bleeding, need attention, but this child's injury will heal on its own.

Go to the Emergency Department

Your one-year-old has just learned to walk. Like all children at that stage, she falls down a lot, especially when she tries to run. This evening she is hurrying around your living room coffee table and stumbles, hitting her head on the corner of the table just above her eye. She is naturally upset afterward, but she is alert. You first hold a clean cloth against the area for five minutes or so to slow the bleeding. Then you have a look at the injury. It is about a half-inch long or so, lies just above her eyebrow, and is oozing blood. You can see skin edges gaping open a bit. What should you do?

Scenarios like this one are extremely common. Lacerations in the upper face from furniture collisions are frequent among toddlers. The immediate treatment, as any first aid manual will tell you, is to place pressure on the wound to stop the bleeding. A clean cloth works well for this. After you bring her to the emergency department, you should expect they will first wash the wound thoroughly and then have a close look at it. One of several kinds of medicine can be used to numb the skin, if necessary. Depending upon what the doctor sees, the laceration might be closed with very fine suture material or with glue. Lacerations like this nearly always heal quickly and well.

Go to the Emergency Department

Your eleven-year-old son is doing some woodworking and the utility knife he is using slips and slices open a two-inch gash on the inside of his forearm. He presses a cloth on it and comes to show it to you. Before looking closely, both of you take the prudent step of sitting down first. For those not used to looking at these injuries, the first glimpse can make you queasy indeed. You cautiously peel back the bloody cloth and see a laceration that gapes apart at its middle. The wound goes right through the skin and you can see yellowish globs of fatty tissue showing. You quickly replace the cloth and appropriately head for the emergency department. What can you and your son expect there?

Standard management of this sort of wound is first to wash it thoroughly with a large amount of dilute salt solution, called *saline*. The doctor will then look at it closely to make sure there are no bits of grit or the like in the wound. She will then most likely numb the skin and close it in layers, bottom to top. This requires two types of suture material: one so-called absorbable (or dissolving) material for the deeper tissues; the other one non-absorbable, for the skin. If there are no injuries to nerves, major blood vessels, or joints, this kind of wound heals just fine. There will be a visible scar. I have one like that on my forearm from just such an injury.

Call 911

You are cooking dinner in the kitchen and your three-year-old is playing on the floor. He is an active child and you watch him carefully out of the corner of your eye. But in spite of your diligence, his curiosity and lightning-quick moves manage to pull a saucepan of hot soup off the stove and onto his lower face and chest. The area is bright red immediately, and you soon see several blisters on his neck. You also notice that his lips are rapidly swelling since some of the soup caught him there. You realize that he has a significant burn, one that needs medical attention. How should you handle this scary situation?

The good news is that burns of this sort heal quite well without leaving permanent scarring or other damage. But this scenario has a particular aspect that should prompt you to call for immediate help: it is possible that the immediate swelling from the burn will affect his breathing by making his airway smaller. Paramedics will know how to handle this possibility on the way to the emergency department.

RASHES

Children have sensitive skin. They also have a higher surface-to-volume ratio, meaning they have relatively more skin than do adults. These facts are a principal reason why children often develop skin rashes. Most parents have had the experience of suddenly noticing a rash on their child, often appearing out of the blue and unaccompanied by any other symptoms. Chapter 10 breaks down rashes into the categories physicians use because those distinctions are key in deciding what a parent should do when their child gets one. Most parents know a simple rash in an otherwise healthy-appearing child does not need attention from a physician in the middle of the night. But there are exceptions to that good general rule; some rashes are signs of serious things. So although most rashes can be managed with watchful waiting, sometimes a phone call to the doctor or even a visit to the emergency department is best. Here are a couple of examples of rashes.

Watchful Waiting

Your second-grade daughter has an itchy nose. She has had a bit of a runny nose for several days from a cold, and she has been diligently blowing her nose as she has been taught. But after a few days of this, her nose is red and raw. It itches, so she has been rubbing it frequently. Now you notice that about a half-inch below her nostrils there is a scabby-looking spot that she has picked open several times. When you look closely at the area, you see some amber-colored, crusting spots oriented as satellites around the bigger scab she has been picking at. What is this, and what should you do about it?

What you are looking at are typical *impetigo* sores. Under the nose is a very common place to see them, another being just outside the lips. There are not very many of them, and most likely you can take care of these at home and then keep an eye on them to make sure they resolve.

Watchful Waiting

Your ten-year-old son has come home at the end of a July day spent on a friend's farm. He is dusty and grimy. He also is itching his thighs and upper arms nearly constantly. You see that he has about ten or twenty raised bumps in those areas. The bumps stick up above his skin surface perhaps a quarter-inch or so. Surrounding several of them are red, blotchy areas that form a sort of halo. The ones he can reach have scratches on them from his itching. He otherwise feels fine. What is this and what should you do about it?

This child has typical *hives*. This case is instructive because much of the time we have no idea what the inciting trigger was. This child has spent a windy day in an environment outside his usual one with multiple potential hive-makers such as grasses and other plants, dusty barns, and animals. The only way to get any clue as to what did this is to see if it happens again and then do some detective work. For this episode, the important thing is that he has no swelling in his mouth, difficulty swallowing, or breathing troubles. You should be able to make your son comfortable and care for him at home.

Call the Doctor

We can modify the above scenario just a little to make calling for advice a good plan. Let us say your son has many, many hives. He still has no airway swelling or breathing troubles, but the itching is driving him crazy. You have given him a dose of diphenhydramine (Benadryl, many others) for the itching (more about how that works in chapter 10), but it does not seem to have helped very much.

In such a situation, it would make sense to call for some advice. We have several medications to block the hive process. Your doctor may want to consider prescribing one of these.

Call the Doctor

Your one-year-old was diagnosed a few days ago with an ear infection after having fever for a day. He is taking amoxicillin (Amoxil, many others), a commonly prescribed oral antibiotic for this problem. Today he is better. His fever is gone, he is eating normally, and he is acting totally himself. But while putting him to bed you notice his chest and abdomen are covered with tiny red bumps. The rash does not seem to be bothering him at all. For example, he is not itching anywhere. What should you do about this?

The answer to this scenario is that his rash is probably from the antibiotic. Although almost any medicine can cause a rash, amoxicillin is notorious for doing this. If your son has no other symptoms than the rash, he does not need to be seen by a doctor. However, depending on how far along your son is in his antibiotic course, many doctors would want to change the antibiotic to another one to complete his treatment for the ear infection. The best thing to do in this scenario is to call the doctor to ask for advice.

Go to the Emergency Department

Your three-year-old daughter has had *upper respiratory infection* (URI) symptoms for a week or so, but she has otherwise seemed herself. She has had no fever, and she does not seem to have any aches or pains. Today she has a rash. The rash feels flat on the skin and consists of tiny purple spots. In a few places, the spots are merging with each other to make larger purplish splotches. It is early evening on a Friday, and you wonder what you should do.

Can this wait until Monday, or should you have her evaluated over the weekend?

If this were your child, the best answer to this scenario is you should take her to the emergency department. Your daughter may have a problem with her blood platelets, such as having too few of them circulating in her blood. You will learn all about this in chapter 10.

Go to the Emergency Department

Your eight-year-old daughter has had a fever as high as 104 degrees all afternoon. She has not complained of anything in particular, but she feels a bit weak and dizzy. In the evening you notice she has a rash on her arms and chest. At first the rash looks like small bites—tiny reddish-purple spots. Over the next couple of hours the rash spreads and the spots seem to be getting a little bigger. She still has a temperature of 104 degrees. She has also become progressively more lethargic and has spent the last three hours asleep on the couch. When you rouse her she seems incoherent, and you are not sure that she even recognizes you. What should you do about this?

The answer here is you should take her to the emergency department. The kind of rash she has can be a sign of a serious illness. Chapter 10 will tell you all about this particular rash, as well as many others, both serious and not.

Call 911

In this scenario we modify the story above in a key way. As the rash progresses, becoming more extensive and coalescing into larger purplish blotches, the child's level of consciousness is also changing. She is becoming progressively more lethargic and has spent the last three hours asleep on the couch. When you rouse her she seems incoherent, and you are not sure that she even recognizes you.

This scenario is best handled with a 911 call for help. Things are moving along quickly and the paramedics will know how to handle the situation. They carry various medications that may be needed to get the child's treatment started.

OVERDOSES, POISONINGS, AND BITES

Children are prone to eat things they should not, sometimes by accident and sometimes on purpose. Sometimes these are medicines, either their own or those of other family members. Other times children, especially toddlers, get into one of the many toxic household products we have under our sinks, in our closets, or in our basements and garages. Even some of the plants around the house or in the yard can be harmful. Insect or animal bites are another way for toxins to enter a child's body.

You should stick on your refrigerator or other prominent place the number of Poison Control: 1-800-222-1222. Make sure everyone in the family knows where to find it, as well as babysitters. This national network has made a huge difference in children's health, and we see many fewer injuries from poisonings than we did before it existed. Doctors use Poison Control to get information too. Although some poisonings are common and we are accustomed to handling them, the range of possibilities is vast. Before Poison Control existed, all we doctors had to help us, besides what we learned in training and from personal experience, were reference books that might or might not give us the information we needed. Now we have the Internet with its useful search engines, which is a vast improvement, but what we really need when we are confronted with an unusual situation or with something we have not seen before is immediate access to real experts, called *toxicologists*. Poison Control gives us that.

Poison Control can give you good advice, but they are not standing there looking at your child—you are. So it is helpful for any parent to have a basic knowledge of which things need immediate attention and which do not. Chapter 11 tells you all about that in detail. For now, here are some useful examples.

Watchful Waiting

Your child is sick with a fever. You and your husband have been giving him ibuprofen (Motrin, many others) every six hours as your doctor recommended. You give him a dose and put him to bed. A half hour later he is fussing in his room and your husband, unaware you have given him the medicine, gives him another full dose. When the two of you discover what has happened, you are unsure what to do. Could the double dose harm him? Should you call Poison Control about this? The answer to this scenario is that you do not need to do anything; ibuprofen has a wide margin of safety, and the overdose will not hurt him.

This provides a good opportunity to discuss the issue of making children vomit when they take something they should not. You will read much more about this issue in chapter 11, but here is the gist of the matter. Until some years ago this was common treatment for any potential poisoning situation. At that time we recommended families keep a medicine that caused vomiting, *syrup of ipecac*, available in the house in case this happened. Ipecac was commonly used in emergency departments as well. I am old enough to recall when we even "pumped the stomach" of a child who had eaten something she should not have.

Research now has clearly shown that the risks of inducing vomiting with syrup of ipecac—for example, the risk of having some of the stomach contents get in the child's airway—are far worse than leaving the medicine in the stomach and doing other things to neutralize it. The more extreme treatment of pumping the stomach does not help much, either, although there still are times in more severe situations when we pass a tube into the stomach of child who has taken a medicine overdose or other toxin. You will learn about those exceptions in chapter 11.

Call the Doctor

Your eighteen-month-old is crawling around in her older brother's room. Like many ten-year-olds' rooms, the place is a mess, with toys scattered across the floor. Some of these are assorted small components to metal and plastic construction kits. Your older child is deeply engrossed in a construction project and does not pay any attention to his little sister. Like most toddlers, your daughter puts almost any new object in her mouth as part of exploring what it is. She reaches for a small metal strut. This attracts your son's attention, and he sees her put it in her mouth. He goes to take it away, but finds it is gone—she has swallowed it. She does not cough or choke, just gets upset for a minute or so, after which she seems fine. Your son brings her to you after the event. What should you do? Anything?

As a general rule, anything sufficiently small for a child to swallow is small enough to pass all the way through the digestive tract and make it out in the stool. The reason calling for advice in this situation is the best course is that what to do depends upon several things, most importantly if the object reached the stomach. If your child does something like this and is clearly uncomfortable afterward, or if she refuses to drink because it hurts, then you should take her to the emergency department because this suggests the object is lodged at the entry to her stomach. But if, like this child, she looks fine, it is a good idea to call your doctor because how to proceed is a judgment call.

Go to the Emergency Department

Your three-year-old daughter manages to climb up to the medicine cabinet above the bathroom sink and grab a bottle of acetaminophen (Tylenol, many others). Although the bottle has a childproof cap, she gets it open somehow. Your ten-year-old son finds his sister sitting on the floor intently picking up the capsules and eating them. He takes them all away and tells you about it when you get home an hour later.

In spite of eating the capsules, your child looks totally fine. You try to figure out how many she took, but you are not sure how many were in the now half-empty bottle. Your son says he found ten or fifteen on the floor. What should you do? Should you watch her for a few hours to see if she gets sick? Should you take her to the emergency department? If you should, can you drive her there yourself or should you call 911 for an ambulance?

The answer to what to do in this scenario is that you should take her to the emergency department. If you were to call Poison Control first, always a good idea, that is what they would advise you to do. But you can take her there yourself because you have some time. What will the doctors do for her there?

Overdoses of acetaminophen are common, and it is well known what to do about them. What many parents do not know is that this drug, although quite safe when used correctly, can cause serious harm when overdosed. The toxic effects are not immediate—they take hours, or even days, to evolve. What matters most is how much your daughter took. It is a common problem for us not to be sure of this, either because the child is too young to tell us or she refuses to say. It is also common not to know how many pills were in the bottle, so counting the ones left, although helpful in figuring out what the maximum number is that the child may have taken, cannot give us a reliable answer.

The way we assess the potential for serious harm from an acetaminophen overdose is to measure the amount of the drug in the child's bloodstream. Once we know this, we have charts that can tell us if the amount is in the toxic range. If it is, we have a very effective antidote that neutralizes the drug. You will learn more details about this in chapter 11.

Call 911

Your family is doing its annual cleaning of the garage. In the bustle of hauling out a year's accumulation of junk, nobody notices, until it is too late, that your two-year-old has been drinking from a jug of windshield washer fluid. As with the scenario above, it is mysterious how he got the childproof cap off—perhaps it was not screwed on all the way—but such things happen. He gets your attention when he starts to cough and sputter, after which he seems to be breathing faster than usual. What should you do? Do you need to bring him to the emergency department? If so, how?

The best thing to do in this scenario is to call 911 for an ambulance ride unless you live very, very close to an emergency department. Among other noxious things, windshield washer fluid contains methanol, which can be quite toxic even in modest amounts. Your son needs prompt, quite possibly emergency, attention.

HEADACHES, CONVULSIONS, AND ALTERED MENTAL STATES

Earlier in the chapter you read some scenarios about head injuries. But children often have problems with their heads other than getting conked on them. As with head injuries, these non-traumatic problems range from the trivial to the life-threatening, and it can be difficult for parents, or even physicians at times, to tell these situations apart. Of course anything involving the brain is worrisome to parents, so a significant number of children who appear in the emergency department are there for such complaints. Chapter 12 will tell you in detail what to do about the most common of these, but here are some scenarios to give you the flavor of the possibilities.

Watchful Waiting

Your twelve-year-old daughter has been getting headaches over the past several months. At first it was just every week or so, but now she has them nearly every day in the late afternoon. This evening she has a particularly bad one, the worst so far. She even vomits a few times at the beginning of the headache. She is well otherwise— no fever, cough, or other symptoms—and she is alert. You are understandably worried about these headaches, and you wonder if you should bring her in to the emergency department to see a doctor tonight. Should you?

The answer to this scenario is that, for tonight, watchful waiting will be fine. But it would be best to take your daughter to the doctor in the next few days for an evaluation of her problem. Chapter 12 will tell you much more about headaches, including which kinds need immediate attention.

Call the Doctor

Your three-year-old son has had a runny nose for a day or two. This afternoon you put him down for a nap. About an hour later you hear an odd noise coming from his room and you go in to check on him. You find him lying on his back in his crib. He is flushed and sweating. He is making jerking motions with his arms and legs. Before you can do anything, the movements stop. Afterward he appears drowsy for a couple of minutes, but after that he is alert. He is crying and upset, and you take his temperature—it is 102 degrees. You give him some ibuprofen, and within forty-five minutes his temperature is normal. He now even looks to be his usual, active self. What should you do?

Your child has had what we call a *febrile seizure*. In chapter 12 you will read about what seizures, or convulsions, are and what we do about them. Toddlers have a particular tendency to have these following a rapid rise in temperature. These seizures are brief, and the child often recovers from them as quickly as your child did. They can be frightening for a parent to witness, but they carry no long-term consequences for the child. Sometimes they need prompt evaluation, but if a child recovers as quickly as your child, it is entirely appropriate to call the doctor for advice. He may well want to see your child within a day or so to discuss things. If the seizure is less typical for a febrile seizure, he may suggest you take your child to the emergency department tonight.

For these reasons, the appropriate course of action for this scenario is to call for advice. However, if your personal situation does not allow for getting prompt medical advice, then it would be entirely appropriate to bring this child to the emergency department.

Go to the Emergency Department

It is dinnertime but your fourteen-year-old son has not come down from his bedroom. He came home from school saying he felt a bit ill and would lie down for a nap. You go up to get him and find him asleep in his bed. When you talk to him he rouses a little bit but is still quite drowsy. You snap on the lights to get a better look at him, and he wants you to turn the lights off again because they hurt his eyes. He says he has a headache, and his neck hurts too. This is unusual for him; he rarely has headaches. You feel his forehead and it feels warm. Your thermometer confirms he has a temperature of 102 degrees. He says the headache has been getting worse over the past couple of hours, and he says he has had very little or nothing to drink all day. What should you do? Should you give him some medicine for his fever and headache and then see how he is in the morning? Or does he need to see a doctor tonight?

The best thing to do for him is to take him to the emergency department now. It would be fine for you to drive him there yourself, but his symptoms suggest he could have meningitis. This is an inflammation of the covering of the brain from an infection. Some of these are caused by viruses, others by bacteria. The latter cases are the most serious and need prompt treatment with antibiotics. He needs to be evaluated tonight for this possibility. Chapter 12 will tell you much more about this not-uncommon pediatric condition.

Call 9 1 1

Your sixteen-year-old daughter has been in her usual state of good health until today. Suddenly, during lunch, she slumps to the floor after making a strange cry. She then proceeds to have a several minutes of shaking of her arms and legs. Her lips also become a bit dusky-colored, and she drools some saliva from the corner of her mouth. Afterward she remains on the floor. She moans a little when you shake her but otherwise does not respond to you. What should you do?

This child has had a serious event, what we call a *grand mal seizure*. At this point there is no way to tell the reason for her seizure, although there are several possibilities. She needs to see a doctor to figure things out. If this were your child, the best way to get her medical attention quickly would be to call 911.

ALLERGIC REACTIONS

All parents have heard of allergies: the body reacts to things in the environment—such as foods, plants, and medicines—with unpleasant symptoms. Generally these reactions are only annoying, but sometimes they can be life-threatening. If parents believe their child is having an allergic reaction, how can they decide what best to do considering this wide range of possibilities? Chapter 13 will tell you all about how allergies work and what doctors do about them, but here are some sample scenarios that demonstrate a few choices.

Watchful Waiting

Your ten-year-old has spent a windy summer weekend visiting his cousins on your brother's farm. When he returns on Sunday evening he has a rash all over his abdomen, chest, and upper arms. It itches quite a bit, and he has been scratching, causing a few scabs here and there. He also has a stuffy nose, but otherwise has no problems breathing—no cough or shortness of breath. He enjoyed the weekend but seems pretty uncomfortable from these symptoms. Should you bring him to the doctor tonight? Should you wait until morning and see if he still has these symptoms? Is there anything you can do tonight to make him feel better?

What has happened to him fits with a reaction to something he encountered on the farm. The possible causes form a long list, everything from plant materials like hay and grass to animal hair and dander. It really does not matter now which of those was the culprit—there are some things you can do to make him feel better. These include washing him and his clothes thoroughly to get rid of residual farm material, giving him an over-the-counter medication to block allergic reactions, and applying an anti-inflammatory cream, also available without prescription, to his itching skin. You will read about these practical measures in detail in chapter 13. The bottom line is you definitely can make him feel better without dragging him to the emergency department tonight. It might, however, be a good idea to call your son's doctor within the next couple of days to discuss having him evaluated, especially if he has similar problems again.

Call the Doctor

Your eight-year-old daughter has had nasal allergies for several years—a chronic runny nose during the late summer and fall. Her doctor has diagnosed her with seasonal plant allergies, since that time of the year is when the pollen count is highest, and she takes cetirizine (Zyrtec) every day during those months. It is August and her symptoms have been a bit worse for the past several days. Tonight she has added a cough to her symptom list. You think she also may be a bit short of breath, although she is not breathing fast. She mainly seems a bit less energetic than usual. What can you do about this? Does she need more allergy medications now? Does her cough mean she needs to see a doctor tonight?

The key to this scenario is the breathing problem. It is possible this child's allergies have progressed beyond just inflaming her nose to involving her lower airways too. If this were your daughter, it would be best to call her doctor for advice and perhaps arrange for an evaluation.

Go to the Emergency Department

Your four-year-old son has been playing in the backyard all morning. He just ran into the house crying, saying that he has been stung by bees. You look at the back of his hand and see it is quite red and swollen from at least one sting. His other forearm is also swollen, and it looks as if several bees stung him there too. That arm is quite swollen from his wrist to his elbow. He continues to cry but does not have any trouble breathing. What should you do?

The doctors in the emergency department will be able to improve your child's symptoms very quickly with various medications. In this situation, it would be reasonable for you to drive your son to the emergency department.

Call 911

Your family is eating out in a restaurant. Your nine-year-old son is curious to try lobster. He would like one of the live ones in the tank at the side of the dining room, but the occasion is not *that* special. He settles for a dish containing bits of lobster in a cream sauce. About fifteen minutes after starting the dinner, he says he feels funny; his lips and tongue feel thick. You also notice his voice seems a bit hoarse, and it sounds as if his breathing is becoming labored and difficult. You tell him to stop eating the dinner, since you appropriately suspect he is developing some sort of reaction to it. Other than that, what should you do? Perhaps give him some water to wash the food down and clear his mouth?

The answer to this one is you should spoil everyone's dinner by pulling out your cell phone and calling 911. He is most likely developing a severe reaction to his dinner, probably the lobster because shellfish is a common allergy. Most of these reactions are mild. But the particular symptoms he is experiencing suggest he is at risk for developing very severe breathing problems very quickly. The medical term for what he is experiencing is *anaphylaxis*—a life-threatening allergic event. He needs attention as soon as possible, and paramedics carry medications to counteract the developing allergic reaction. These medications are very effective, and the odds are overwhelming your son will be fine. After this episode is over, though, and you have gone home from the emergency department, you should take him to the doctor for an evaluation and a discussion about how to prevent this problem in the future. Chapter 13 will tell you what this entails.

This chapter has been a whirlwind tour, a sampling of what you will learn in the rest of the book. As you have read, all the categories of medical problems children develop contain a wide range of possibilities, from the trivial to the very severe. All parents want to find a commonsense middle ground between one of falsely pooh-

poohing symptoms that need emergency department evaluation and one of hyper-anxious over-vigilance that leads to useless (and expensive) midnight trips to the doctor. The way to achieve that balance is to understand how doctors look at all these common symptoms, how we sort out the serious from the not serious. This book is emphatically *not* intended to encourage you to practice medicine on your children, and nothing can substitute for a physician's evaluation. *However*, there are many practical approaches any parent can learn and understand about how we doctors think and make decisions. Armed with this knowledge, many times you can keep your child from being one of the third of all American children who visit the emergency department each year. But if you do go, understanding how the place is organized and how doctors evaluate common symptoms will tell you what you should expect, and what should happen. This will allow you to advocate for your child to get the best care.

3

FEVER

For thousands of years doctors thought fever was a disease in itself. This was still true even until little more than a century ago. Physicians devised elaborate classifications of fever that they believed distinguished fevers from each other—how high the fever was, how long the fever lasted, if it was constant or if it came and went. They thought each of these various kinds of fever patterns represented different disease processes. Today we know this is not so. Fever is not a disease. It is a sign of disease, a response of the body to a wide variety of things.

Compared with adults, children beyond the age of newborns get a lot of fevers. One reason for this is that a common cause of fever is viral infection, and children get a lot of those as their young bodies encounter all the viruses our adult bodies are accustomed to already. Not only do children get a lot of fevers, but when they do get one, it is often higher than an adult would experience in the same situation. So parents are often confronted with the problem of what to do about it. Fever is usually a harmless thing, although it can make a child uncomfortable; but it also can be a sign of a serious problem that needs prompt medical attention. How can parents tell the difference between these possibilities? The key is to think about fevers in the way doctors do, and this chapter will help you learn how to do that. But first, it helps to understand where fever comes from and how the body makes its temperature go up and down.

The body controls its temperature quite closely. It keeps its internal temperature within a very narrow range in spite of a wide variety of external conditions. How does it do that? The easiest way to think about it is to remember that the body has, up in the brain, a thermostat similar to the one connected to the furnace in your house. The sensor in the brain thermostat constantly monitors the temperature in the blood flowing by it and adjusts the body's temperature up or down to return to the set point for the thermostat. If the blood temperature is too low, the body conserves heat; if the blood temperature is too high, the body dumps heat.

Where does internal body heat come from? The body is not unlike the engine in your car. For that matter, it even resembles a simple fire. Like an engine or a fire, the body uses oxygen to burn fuel to produce energy and as a result gives off heat, carbon dioxide, and water. Of course it does not use flames to do this; instead, it uses chemical reactions. Looking at it this way explains why, in common with all creatures, we need oxygen—all combustion requires the oxygen present in air. It also explains why major components of the air we breathe out are carbon dioxide and water vapor, because these are the normal byproducts of combustion, of burning. We get rid of them by breathing them out.

The fuel for our internal fire comes in the form of the food we eat, and we can measure that fuel in *calories*. In chemistry and physics, the calorie is a unit of heat. We store fuel between meals and "burn" it when we need it using a complex series of chemical reactions. Many of us worry about eating too many calories, because if we eat far more than we burn away, we store the excess fuel as fat. The way a dietician knows a particular food has a certain number of calories is that, if measured in a laboratory, the amount of chemical energy stored in the food will give off a specific amount of heat when burned. The precise scientific definition of a calorie is the amount of heat needed to raise one gram of water by one degree centigrade.

What does all this have to do with fever? Fever is about regulating the temperature of the body, and it uses the heat generated from the body's internal combustion engine to do this. Under normal circumstances, body heat is more than enough for the brain's thermostat to work with. But not always. An example of an abnormal situation when the body's heat production would not be enough for its needs would be if you were sitting in subzero weather for hours without a coat.

We adjust our body's temperature in several ways. The most important of them is through our blood circulation, which in this instance you can think of as similar to a household heating system that uses water circulating throughout the house in pipes. Heat radiates away from our body surface, so by directing blood toward or away from our skin we can unload or conserve heat. The pipes of our blood vessels have a delicate system of control gates to accomplish this task.

This is why someone who has been exercising vigorously looks flushed; the exercise has generated excess heat, and the blood vessels of the skin, especially the face, become engorged with blood to help unload the heat that came from the fuel burned during the exercise. It is also why someone who is cold will look pale; the body conserves heat by redirecting as much blood as possible away from the body surface. If a swing in blood flow inward to raise our temperature happens very fast, we respond by shivering. This is why we shiver if we go outside without a coat in the winter; our bodies are redirecting blood flow from our skin to our core in order to maintain temperature.

Once you understand this dynamic of how the body conserves or releases heat you can also understand how the system might work a little differently in children. If you compare a child's body with an

adult one, you see several differences. For understanding temperature control, the key difference is that the proportion of a child's
body that is on the surface to that on the inside, called the surface-
to-volume ratio, is higher than that of an adult. We adults have
much more of our bulk inside us compared to the amount we ex-
pose to the world. With this is mind, it is not at all surprising that a
child's temperature is a lot more variable than is an adult's. This is
particularly so in infants. With their small bodies, normal infants
may not be able to conserve enough heat to keep their body temperatures up even in a room of normal temperature. Premature infants
almost always need extra warmers to keep their temperature in the
right spot.

There is one other thing that is important for understanding body
temperature control: it varies in a predictable way during the day.
On average, body temperature is a degree or so higher in the evening than it is early in the morning. This is partly because of the
actions of several hormones that affect the brain thermostat and that
are unrelated to fevers. But it is also because of our internal heat
production. When we are active, moving about and using our fuel-
burning and heat-generating muscles, average core temperature
rises. This reaches a peak in the evening. Then we go to bed and
fuel-burning goes down, reaching its lowest point in the middle of
the night.

A key point to know for a parent holding a thermometer in her
child's mouth in the middle of the night is how doctors define the
threshold for fever. It is true individuals can vary from one another
in what is normal for them—some people have temperatures slightly higher than the average, some lower. So what is a fever in me
may not be a fever in you. Where you measure temperature also
matters. Core temperature, such as taken of a child with a rectal
thermometer, is usually a degree or so higher than a simultaneous
measurement taken in the mouth, on the forehead, or under the arm.
As a practical matter, most doctors choose a number that is high

enough so that individual variability and location do not matter. Most choose a value of 100.4 degrees Fahrenheit, or 38 degrees centigrade, as an indication of fever. It is not a perfect answer, but it is a number that has stood the test of time in practice.

So much for heat production and fever. Now we should talk a little about the brain thermostat and what controls it. I have told you it works like the sensor of your furnace to keep temperature at a preset point, and that fever happens when something cranks up the thermostat to a higher setting. What does that and why?

By far the most common cause of fever in children is infection. This is less the case in adults. It is still true for adults that the majority of fevers are caused by infection, but there are many other things that can do it as well. It is more accurate to say that fever, both in adults and children, comes from inflammation, and infection is the most common cause of inflammation.

Inflammation is the intricate system the body uses to react to a vast array of challenges and insults. When you hit your thumb with a hammer and the thumb swells and throbs, that is inflammation. When you accidentally rub a poison ivy leaf on your skin and your skin then itches and blisters, that is inflammation too. And when germs invade your son's ear and cause an ear infection, the tiny space inside his ear becomes very inflamed indeed. All of these things can lead to the cardinal signs and symptoms of inflammation: pain, swelling, redness, and increased warmth. The substances that cause these signs also cause fever.

The fever-inducing substances belong to a family of molecules called *cytokines*. Cytokines are released by specialized body cells in certain circumstances, such as injury or invasion by germs. You can think of cytokines as the body's "first responder" cells that rush to any threatened area. Once they get there they act as all good first responders do: before they go into action, they first call for more help. They then go to work. They attack any invaders they find, such as germs. When they finish that task, they work to clean up the mess infection leaves behind.

It is these messages, the cytokine distress calls, which travel throughout the bloodstream and reset the brain's thermostat. Germs themselves can also release substances that have the same effect on the brain. The sudden rises and drops a parent often sees in their child's temperature when the child has an infection reflect the usually brief time cytokines are in the blood. Sustained fever for many hours can happen if these materials are steadily present.

Since fever is not a disease by itself but is rather a sign of other things, the important thing about fever is what it can mean, what it can show about related events in the body. That is what a parent needs to consider when deciding what to do, ranging from nothing to calling 911. But before we examine those possibilities and how a doctor decides between them, we should consider that most parents are also concerned by the possibility that fever itself, no matter what the cause, can harm their child. Is that possible?

The short answer is no, fever in itself is not harmful. There are rare exceptions to this when a fever gets extremely high—105 degrees or more—for sustained periods of time. But those are very rare situations that only happen when the child has something intrinsically wrong with her brain thermostat. There is a common situation, however, in which fever can cause trouble in the way the body responds to it. Toddlers are prone to develop brief seizures, or convulsions, if their body temperature rises very fast. So-called febrile seizures are seen in 1 to 2 percent of all normal children, and the propensity to get them tends to run in families. Febrile seizures in themselves have no long-standing consequences, but if your child is prone to them, fever control is important. You will read much more about febrile seizures in chapter 12, which covers problems with the brain and nervous system.

Although fever causes no harm to a child's body, it certainly can make a child uncomfortable. Long ago many doctors believed fever had beneficial effects for helping a child combat infections, but we now know there is no reason not to treat a fever if doing so will make the child more comfortable. In other words, you will not affect your child's ability to fight an infection by treating the fever. On the other hand, if your child has a fever and looks and acts fine with it, there is no compelling reason to give medicine for the fever just because your child's temperature is up. (Like most things in medicine, there is an important exception to this principle—infants with fever. You will read about that later in the chapter.)

There are two effective drugs to treat fever—acetaminophen (Tylenol, many others) and ibuprofen (Motrin, many others). Both are available without prescription. The dose to use is written on the box, but those suggested doses are often based on a child's age. Doctors, knowing that children of the same age come in different sizes, base the doses on weight. Many although not all products give both the age and weight ranges. For acetaminophen, the dose is about 5–6 milligrams per pound, given as needed as often as every four hours; for ibuprofen, the dose is about 4–5 milligrams per pound, given as needed as often as every six hours.

Although these medicines are unrelated chemically, they both work in a similar fashion to lower fever by resetting the brain's central thermostat back toward normal. They only work for a few hours, though, so if your child continues to have fever-causing cytokines circulating in the bloodstream, his fever could go back up again. You can then repeat the dose at the intervals noted above.

All this scientific background information about fever may be interesting, but it does not much help answer a parent's questions: What do I do about this particular fever in my child right now? Should I worry? Should I call someone or bring my child to the emergency department? The answer to these questions is a bit maddening. It is an answer doctors give a lot, which is this: It depends. To understand what it depends upon, and to help you make that important decision, we can go back to the four scenarios from chapter 2 and look at them a bit closer. I will repeat them to refresh your memory.

WATCHFUL WAITING

Your four-year-old son has had a runny nose for a couple of days, but this has not seemed to affect him very much. He is still active and playful, and he is eating normally. Today you notice he coughs occasionally, but he does not seem short of breath or otherwise bothered by the cough. When you are giving him his evening bath you notice he feels a bit warm, so you take his temperature—it is 101.5 degrees. He still seems normal otherwise except for the runny nose and cough. What should you do?

The key point in this scenario is that the fever needs to be put in the context of how the child is doing overall. He is alert, acting himself, and not complaining of anything. He has some cold symptoms, but these do not appear to be bothering him much. This is common. In general, children with colds tolerate the annoying symptoms of cough and runny nose a lot better than adults with the same infection do. This is a good thing because children, especially toddlers, get a large number of colds. Some research says one cold per month is the average for a young child who spends a lot of time with other children. You will read much more about colds and other examples of what we call *upper respiratory infections* in the next chapter. Just now we are concentrating on the fever and what to do about it.

What this scenario boils down to is this: does the mere presence of the fever make you think your child needs medical attention in the night? After all, he is not acting any differently. You only took his temperature on a whim and were surprised to discover he even had an elevated temperature.

The answer about what to do in this scenario is what we have been calling *watchful waiting*, a fancy term for just waiting to see what happens, to see if anything changes. You do not need to call anybody, and your son certainly does not need to be seen by a doctor tonight. What would make you change your mind about that plan? A good approach would be to call the doctor or have your son seen if he has persistent fever for twenty-four hours or so, or if he gets additional symptoms, things like worsening cough or a new pain in his ears or throat.

There is no reason not to treat his fever with either of the medicines you read about earlier, but truth to tell, he could well not notice the difference. Many children do not seem to mind fever at all. When parents give them medicine for it, the parents are often treating themselves as much as they are the child. But many children do act listless with a fever, and for them it can be useful to treat the increased temperature. This lets you see how your child acts when the fever improves. It is very reassuring to have a droopy or even lethargic child perk up when their temperature comes down. As you will read, a child with a fever who is also disoriented and lethargic is one of the signs that things are potentially more serious.

CALL THE DOCTOR

Your eight-year-old daughter is in the third grade. She was well until yesterday, when she came home from school looking a bit droopy and complaining of a headache. She did not eat much for dinner, and afterward she went right to bed, something unusual for her. You cannot sleep much yourself because you are worried about her, so in the middle of the night you go into her room to see how she is doing. She awakens easily and feels warm on her forehead so you take her temperature—it is 103 degrees. You ask how she feels. She replies she has a mild headache and a sore, scratchy throat. She also has a stomach ache. You turn on the light to get a better look at her. Her cheeks are flushed but otherwise she looks okay. What should you do?

One thing to notice is that this child does not have symptoms of a cold, such as congestion and a runny nose. A school-age child with a cold does not need to see a doctor. Another thing to notice is that she complains of a headache and a sore throat. This combination is a common one when a child has strep throat—an infection by bacteria with the long scientific name of *Streptococcus pyogenes*. This type of infection needs treatment with antibiotics, but not tonight. If your daughter has strep, there is no good evidence that getting out of bed at two in the morning to bring your child to the emergency department to get antibiotics for the strep, rather than waiting until the next day, will make the strep get better any faster. And not all sore throats are strep. Many are caused by viruses, for which there is no specific treatment.

There is another important aspect of this case to consider, and that is the headache and lethargy. As you will learn in a later chapter, serious infection around the brain, called *meningitis*, can begin like this. The things that make meningitis extremely unlikely in this case are the mildness of the headache and the fact that the child is alert and appropriate when you wake her up. She also lacks an important sign of meningitis, which is a sore and stiff neck, best identified by an inability to touch the chin to the chest.

This particular fever scenario is a little more complicated than the first one. It is fever with some other significant things. If this were your child, you would benefit from getting a little advice. How severe is the sore throat? How bad is the headache? Can she eat and swallow liquids normally? So a reasonable course here would be to call your doctor for help in sorting things out. Depending upon your circumstances, that could certainly be the next morning if your daughter is not better.

GO TO THE EMERGENCY DEPARTMENT

You have a three-week-old daughter. She has been fine since you brought her home from the hospital at two days of age, and she was fine when she saw the doctor last week for a well-baby checkup. This evening you put her down in her crib after a feeding. When you go in to get her several hours later, you notice she feels warm to you so you take her temperature and find it is 102 degrees. She may be a bit fussier than usual and her nose is a little stuffy, but overall she does not appear to have anything in particular wrong with her—just the fever. What should you do?

This scenario is different because it involves an infant; that is the key. Your daughter is perhaps a little fussy, but otherwise she looks fine except for the fever. In particular, she has been feeding well and has been alert. So she is a lot like the boy in the first scenario who looked to be his normal self except for some mild cold symptoms. Why should we not use a strategy of watchful waiting on this infant? After all, it seems like the same situation.

The answer is that infants are a special case. Their immune systems, the cells in the body whose job it is to fight off infection, are not completely mature yet. It will be several months at least before they are. This means babies cannot ward off invading germs as well as older children can. So we must be extra vigilant about protecting them from that possibility. One way we do that is to be extra careful in how we deal with babies with fevers. Some babies, ones who are extremely ill from infection, cannot even mount a fever, so the absence of fever in an infant who looks very ill does not eliminate the possibility of infection. This child is not that sick, however. She just has a fever and a bit of a stuffy nose.

A related disadvantage infants have is that when an infection is present, they can become seriously ill much quicker than do older children or adults. The bodies of older people can put up a good battle against a serious infection for many hours. Infants cannot reliably do that. Their immature immune systems put up a much more feeble fight against invading germs, allowing the germs to gain the upper hand rapidly. A baby can go from looking fine to being critically ill in a matter of hours. A plan of watchful waiting for a baby with fever thus can be dangerous. How dangerous?

If your baby is in a situation like this scenario—having a fever without much else and generally looking good—you should be reassured that in the great majority of cases your baby will be fine. The chances are still low that a dangerous infection is present. But the point is we cannot take a chance because babies are not fully equipped to fight off infection; we have to help them. The way doctors treat infants with fevers is well established. If an infant less than two months of age has a temperature of 100.4 degrees or more the baby needs an examination by a doctor and nearly always some laboratory tests to see if there is any evidence of infection.

The most important of these tests use samples of several body fluids to see if there are bacteria present. The problem is that these tests, called *cultures*, take at least two days to yield a result. That is because the way a culture works is to take a sample of each body fluid and put it in nutrient broth, or food for bacteria, and then to put the broth in an incubator. If there are bacteria present, they will grow and multiply in the broth. We cannot identify a few bacteria because they are so small. Once they multiply in the broth, however, we can see them and identify what kind they are. But that process takes time. The resulting practical problem is that while the cultures are incubating, the doctor does not know if the baby has a serious infection or not. By the time the culture results are back, the baby could be dangerously ill from the infection. We need to prevent that from happening and protect the baby.

The safest way to handle this problem is to treat the baby with antibiotics until the culture results come back. If the results are negative—no growth of bacteria—then the antibiotics can be stopped. If bacteria do grow, we have a head start on the situation and we continue the medicine. We know from experience that oral antibiotics will not do the job in this situation; the medicine needs to go directly into the circulation, which means the baby needs to come into the hospital and have a tiny plastic tube placed in one of the veins of the hand, foot, or scalp. This tube is called an *intravenous line*, or IV for short. This entire process is known in doctor jargon as a *sepsis workup* (or *sepsis rule out*), since *sepsis* is the medical term for bacteria in the bloodstream.

There are three body fluids where infection could be hiding: the blood, the urine, or the spinal fluid, the clear fluid in which floats the brain and spinal cord. The last of these is potentially the most serious, and babies have a particular propensity to have bacteria that are circulating in the blood break out of the bloodstream and invade the spinal fluid, causing an infection termed *meningitis*. Depending upon the circumstances, and there is an element of physician judgment involved, the child may not need all three cultures done. But for a complete and thorough sepsis workup, all three fluids need to be sampled. To get the blood sample, we use a small needle inserted into a vein; to get the urine, we use a tiny plastic tube passed up into the bladder; to get the spinal fluid, we place a small needle into the space within the spinal column. The last is called a *lumbar puncture*, or *spinal tap*.

A spinal tap seems to most parents to be a frightening thing. After all, we are putting a needle between the bones of the back, and everybody knows the spinal cord is in there somewhere. But the procedure really is not dangerous at all, and the size of the needle is the same as the one used to take a blood sample. Further, the needle is going into a fluid-filled sack that is well below the spinal cord itself. We also get useful information from the spinal fluid even before the culture is completed because infection, if it is present, generally causes to be present inflammatory cells we can see through the microscope, cells that would not be there in normal circumstances. So the test gives important information right away to help answer the key question: Does this baby have an infection?

This fever scenario is a special case—an infant with fever. There are other times, though, when the best course of action is to take a child who is older than a baby to the emergency department in the middle of the night for evaluation of a fever. What are the guiding principles for making that kind of decision?

The most important principle is the one physicians use: what else is there besides the fever, that is, how does the child look and act? Serious infection is the main concern. Children with such an infection look sick. They might be confused or disoriented, be difficult to awaken, or they might respond poorly when you talk to them. They often have pale, pasty, or mottled skin. A child with an unserious fever is often uncomfortable and cranky, but these symptoms usually improve if you bring the fever down with medicine. Parents know their child the best. If your child with fever looks not right to you, then the best course is to bring them to the doctor for an evaluation, no matter what the hour is.

This chapter is about what to do with fever, mostly in isolation from other findings. As you will read in coming chapters, another reason to bring your child to the emergency department is if the fever is accompanied by other things, such as painful or swollen areas of an arm or a leg, a severe cough, or severe abdominal pain. There are useful principles parents can put into practice about how to evaluate those things too. and you will learn all about them in later chapters.

CALL 911

Your two-year-old son has been cranky with a fever all afternoon. You gave him some acetaminophen (Tylenol, many others) for the fever and it seemed to help. This evening, though, he did not eat anything at all for dinner and seemed more listless. You put him in his crib and then go to check on him a couple of hours later. He feels hot to your touch, so he clearly has a fever again. What bothers you more than his fever is that he does not respond to you at all, even when you pick him up. He is limp as a dishcloth. His complexion is washed out, even grey-appearing. His breathing is very shallow; as you watch him there are moments when you wonder if he is breathing at all. When you shake him a little he only moans. What should you do?

This chapter's final scenario illustrates some of the principles we have been discussing. This boy has a fever. More importantly, he is unresponsive, limp, and has a mottled and pasty complexion. He appears to have some pauses in his breathing. Those things would be troubling even if he did not have a fever. When we combine those symptoms with his high temperature, it's clear he has a significant chance of being extremely ill. He may well soon develop worse problems with his breathing—it could even completely stop. So he needs to reach medical care quickly. Your best course of action here is to call 911 for help. The paramedics will bring medicines and equipment to start treatment even before your child gets to the emergency department.

CHECKLIST AND ACTION PLANS FOR FEVER

We will end this chapter, as we will all of the following chapters, with a checklist to help you decide what to do. It sums up the chapter in a nutshell. The goal is for you to assess the situation as a doctor does, looking for the key items a doctor uses to decide what to do. There are four options, ranging from doing little or nothing to calling for immediate help. A good way to use the list is like this: if you are unsure of what you are seeing, move your action plan up a notch to the next level.

Watchful Waiting

1. The fever does not affect your child's behavior much.
2. Your child is still drinking fluids.
3. The fever improves with acetaminophen or ibuprofen.
4. There may be mild additional symptoms, such as cough, but no more than that.

Call the Doctor

1. The fever does not get better with acetaminophen or ibuprofen.
2. There are moderate additional symptoms that persist, such as cough or sore throat.
3. Your child is not drinking fluids well.

Take Your Child to the Emergency Department

1. Your child is two months of age or less.
2. Your child is not drinking fluids at all.
3. There are prominent additional symptoms, such as severe cough or breathing troubles.
4. Your child is not acting right; for example, your child is listless, lethargic, or confused.

Call 911

1. Your child does not respond to you.
2. There are severe additional symptoms, such as gasping for breath or convulsions.

4

COUGHS, SNEEZES, SORE THROATS, AND EARACHES

What physicians call *upper respiratory infections*, or URIs, afflict a large portion of the children sitting in emergency department waiting rooms. This is unfortunate, because the great majority of these children do not need to be there. This is because most URIs do not need any treatment at all. For those few that do, the treatment can nearly always wait until the next day. This chapter will help you decide which group your child is in.

Of course the parents sitting in the emergency department waiting room are not there because they want to be; rather, they are just trying to do the right thing for their child, like all parents. In my experience, the vast majority of these parents are well aware their child is not seriously ill. Their main concern is that the URI is more than a simple cold, or is possibly on the verge of worsening into something more serious. These are reasonable concerns. What you will learn in this chapter is how doctors decide if either of those things are happening. We will not be talking here about more substantial breathing problems, such as wheezing and difficulty in taking a breath—those more-serious issues are for the next chapter. This one is about sore throats, runny noses, and earaches.

The first thing to know about URIs is that the majority of them are caused by viruses. These are small bits of genetic material encased in an envelope of protein. They are so tiny—far smaller than bacteria—that they cannot be seen under a standard microscope; they can only be observed using an extremely powerful electron microscope. Viruses are not really alive in the sense we usually mean because by themselves they cannot reproduce and make more viruses. They really cannot do anything at all until they infect one of our body's cells. Here is how that process works.

We can become infected by a virus when it gets introduced into our bodies. For the viruses that cause URIs, this entry takes place through our mouth, nose, or sometimes our eyes. The invasion can happen in several ways. Someone already infected with the virus can sneeze in our face, sending a cloud of droplets of nasal or oral fluids flying through the air. These secretions are loaded with viral particles that we breathe in, after which they land on the tissues of our upper respiratory tract. More common, though, is for respiratory viruses to pass from person to person through touch. A person who is infected with a virus often has viral particles on his hands that get there via handling tissues used to blow his nose or from touching infected mucous in his nose. An itchy nose gets scratched, transferring viral particles to the fingers. When the infected person touches someone without the infection, the virus can then jump to the new host. This is why simply washing your hands and properly disposing of virus-contaminated tissues is the single most important way to reduce the spread of respiratory viruses.

Once on the tissues of a new person's body, such as on the lining of the nose, the virus attaches itself to the cells there. Within a few hours the virus is absorbed inside the body cells and immediately begins to cause mischief. The protective packaging envelope of the virus dissolves, and the viral genetic material is released. When that happens, the virus takes over the normal internal cellular machinery and diverts it from its normal functions to one of becoming a factory for making new viruses. It is a sort of cellular hijacking. After a time the infected cells burst open, releasing a microscopic cloud of new viral particles, which then infect other nearby cells, ramping up the infection. When enough cells have been infected, a process that generally takes several days, the newly infected person begins to feel the symptoms of the infection.

These symptoms can include fever, although not everybody with a URI gets a high temperature. If they do, it is because the virus stimulates the body to release some of those substances you learned about in chapter 3 that reset the brain's thermostat. The viral infection inflames the tissues in the area, causing the boggy, red noses and scratchy throats with which we are all familiar. It also causes the infected areas to increase their production of mucous, leading to a runny nose and excess mucous in the back of the throat. The inflammation irritates the nose and throat, causing soreness and a cough. The excess mucous also contributes to the cough.

If you were a virus, your goal would be to manufacture as many offspring viral particles as possible and through them to infect others, perpetuating the cycle and contributing to the overall survival of the virus in the world. But a respiratory virus has to work fast because it usually does not get much time to accomplish this; as soon as the infection starts, the body's immune system mobilizes its troops first to contain and then to eliminate the invaders. In fact, the inflammation and increased mucous are key parts of the tools the body uses to do this. The inflammation brings infection-fighting cells to the scene, and the mucous helps wash away the viral particles. It also washes away all the lining cells destroyed by the virus, plus a good number of the body's spent infection-fighting cells, which is why the mucous typically goes from clear and runny to cloudy and thick as the URI progresses. Within a few days the virus is eliminated and the tissues return to normal. But there may be aftereffects, which you will read about in the next chapter.

Every child gets a lot of URIs. Their young bodies spend the first few years of their lives meeting the many respiratory viruses with which we share our world, and their immune systems need practice in how to respond to them. Since viral infections are so common in children, children are exposed to viruses frequently, especially at daycare, preschool, and school. Toddlers share cookies and toys that have been chewed on by a playmate, for example. The result is that the average preschooler gets anywhere from six to twelve URIs each year.

We have no effective therapy to kill URI viruses, so there is no specific treatment. In particular, antibiotics, which kill bacteria, have no effect on viruses. Most parents know this, but the urge to want antibiotics just in case there is an early bacterial infection brewing is a strong one. This urge needs to be resisted.

If most parents know that URIs are viral and typically mild, why do more than a few bring their child to the emergency department? What can worry parents enough that they bring their child in is the concern that the viral URI might progress to something worse. This is not an unreasonable fear because it happens. There are several common examples of the phenomenon, and understanding them will help you decide what to do with your sneezing, coughing child in the middle of the night.

By far the most common complication of a viral URI is an acute middle ear infection—termed *acute otitis media*—although this is quite dependent upon age. Children between the ages of about six months and two years of age account for the great majority of ear infections. Not surprisingly, this is also the age group that accounts for a huge number of URIs in childhood—the two are linked. Over three-quarters of all children will have at least one ear infection by the age of two, and a third of children will have six or more episodes of ear infection by the time they are five years old. Some children are particularly prone to getting them. In fact, ear infection is the most commonly diagnosed disease in all of childhood. Inevitably a good portion of the children waiting to see the emergency department doctor are there because they have an ear infection. Do they all need to be there? Do any of them need to be there? Before we can answer that question, we need to talk a little more about what causes an ear infection.

What we refer to here as an ear infection is actually an infection of just one part of the ear, called the *middle ear*. When a doctor looks into your child's ear using an *otoscope*, the technical term for the small tube with a light on the end and a magnifying glass on the front, he is looking at the ear drum, a translucent patch of skin that sits at the end of the blind alley that is the ear canal. On the other side of the ear drum is the middle ear. The job of the middle ear is to transmit sounds to the brain. It does this in a very ingenious way.

The middle ear is filled with air. It gets this air via a connecting tube, called the *Eustachian tube*, that runs from the middle ear to the back of the nose. You can feel the function of the tube every time you go up or down in altitude, such as flying in a plane or driving in the mountains; you feel a popping sensation as air either leaves the middle ear when you go up or flows back into the cavity when you go down. There are three tiny bones that span the space inside the middle ear between the back side of the ear drum and the sensing mechanism of the brain. When sound hits the ear drum, the drum vibrates. The tiny bones that span the middle ear then themselves vibrate in succession and transmit the motion of what first bounced off the ear drum to the brain's sensor, which sits on the other side of the middle ear. This sensor transmits the signal to the brain, and the result is what we perceive as sound.

The middle ear is normally sterile, or free of all germs. But it is connected by the Eustachian tube to the back of the nose, which is teeming with germs. The distance from nose to middle ear is quite short. How does the body keep germs from crawling up the tube and getting into the middle ear?

The answer is that the ear has several ingenious defenses to keep that from happening. The main protection is a mechanical one. The Eustachian tube is lined with cells coated with tiny hair-like projections. On top of these hairs (called *cilia*) there is normally a thin layer of mucous. The hairs all beat and wave in unison, which under the microscope looks like a bed of kelp plants waving together on the sea floor or football fans doing the wave at a game. As the cilia do this, they drive the mucous layer down from the middle ear to the nose. The effect is like a conveyer belt. Any bacteria that make it into the lower reaches of the Eustachian tube are swept neatly out the door and back into the nose.

It is a wonderfully efficient system, but it is also one immediately vulnerable to any process that interferes with it. The bacteria are always waiting, ready to pounce if there is any breakdown in the mucous conveyer belt. The most common cause of such a breakdown is a viral URI.

When a virus attacks the cells lining the nose and throat, causing the familiar runny nose and scratchy throat, it also affects the cells in and near the Eustachian tube. When that happens, the mucous turns from its normal thin, clear state to thick and cloudy, which can easily clog the tube. There is also swelling around the opening of the tube, which can close it off. In addition, when the lining cells of the lower part of the tube become infected, many of them are shed off. Those remaining no longer have their cilia beat in the nice, uniform manner that made the conveyer-belt system work. So germs now can manage to make the journey from the nose to the normally germ-free middle ear.

Once the germs get to the middle ear, they reproduce and quickly reach great numbers. It takes a typical germ only twenty to thirty minutes to divide into two germs, which then themselves divide, and so on until the middle ear is stuffed with germs. The infection draws the body's normal disease-fighting cells to the scene. The subsequent battle between germs and body cells produces many casualties—dead germs and cells—that, along with all the mucous, further fills the middle ear with fluid. Remember that normally the middle ear has little to no fluid in it, being filled with air. All the fluid raises the pressure in the middle ear, bulges the ear drum out the wrong way, and thereby causes pain. When the doctor looks down the ear canal of a child with a middle ear infection, he sees a red, inflamed, sore, and bulging ear drum; all these things are the hallmarks of otitis media. The most common trigger for this chain of events is the viral URI that interfered with the middle ear's normal housekeeping functions.

As you read earlier, ear infections are the most common diagnosis made by doctors of a sick child. So they are a rite of passage for nearly all children, and some children get quite a lot of them. They can lead to more-serious infection, although that is rare. One potential problem is if the bacteria in the middle ear escape from there and make it into the bloodstream, circulating throughout the body. If that happens, the circulating germs can settle out in some other body organ and cause infection there. Depending upon which organ that is, the results can be serious indeed. But again, that is a very rare occurrence.

The middle ear bacteria can also cause problems in the immediate area surrounding the middle ear by breaking out from there and invading the nearby tissues. Although it is uncommon, the bacteria can infect what are called the *mastoid air cells*. These are hollow cavities within the bone behind the ear. You can feel your mastoid bone if you put your finger behind your ear; it is the hard bump just behind the ear cartilage. The condition is called *mastoiditis*, and it may even need both antibiotics and surgery to cure, although such surgery is very uncommon these days with the powerful antibiotics we have.

If ear infections can cause serious complications, is it crucial they be treated right away with antibiotics? If you believe your child might have an ear infection, should you come to the emergency department right away to get him evaluated? The answer is that recent research has shown immediate treatment is not crucial. In fact, not all ear infections need to be treated. The body's local defenses in the region often can clear the infection on their own. Ear infection does cause a child a lot of pain, which comes from the pressure inside the cavity of the middle ear caused by the buildup of infected fluid. If your child's ear hurts, you can give acetaminophen (Tylenol, many others) or ibuprofen (Motrin, many others) for the pain, but you do not necessarily need to rush to the emergency department to get an antibiotic prescription. The research also has shown that delaying antibiotic treatment for a day does not affect how fast the ear heals.

The common practice in this country (although not everywhere—Europe, for example) has long been to treat all acute ear infections with antibiotics. But we now know that another reasonable approach is to wait a day or so to see if the symptoms get better on their own without antibiotics. Parents have an important role in making this choice. If you and the doctor decide to wait on antibiotic treatment, you can still treat fever and pain with acetaminophen or ibuprofen in the doses listed in the last chapter. There is also available a numbing ear drop that, when dripped down the ear canal onto the ear drum, directly relieves the pain there.

If you think about it, this newer understanding of the natural history of ear infections makes sense. Children have been contracting ear infections for many thousands of years, yet we have only had antibiotics for three-quarters of a century. The overwhelming majority of those children in the pre-antibiotic era must have recovered from the infection on their own.

You may have noticed that above I used the weasel words "not necessarily" in my statement regarding whether or not ear infections need prompt evaluation. There are a few times that they do. How can you know when that is? The answer is to look at your child in light of what else she is doing. She will have a fever and probably be fussy. But if she is alert, drinking fluids, and looks good otherwise, you can safely put off having her evaluated. On the other hand, if she is lethargic, glassy-eyed, and not taking fluids, then you should bring her in because those kinds of symptoms can be indicative of a more-serious condition. If you decide to wait and see how your child does before bringing her to the doctor, how much time should you give it? Twenty-four hours is a reasonable amount of time to wait to see if the fever and pain resolve. If they do not, then it would be appropriate to bring your child to the doctor.

URIs can cause other complications besides ear infections. One of them is infection of the sinuses, called *sinusitis*. The sinuses are air-filled cavities in the skull. The largest, called the *maxillary sinuses*, are behind the cheekbones and under the eyes. Others lie behind the nose. Adults have sinuses above the eyes, but these are not developed yet in small children. The sinuses are all lined with cells similar to those found in the middle ear. Like the middle ear, each sinus is connected with the nasal passage via a short tube. Also like the middle ear, the sinuses are normally free of germs, and they stay that way using a similar mechanism of cells with cilia on their surface constantly moving along a mucous layer to exit the sinus into the nasal passage. As with an ear infection, a URI disrupts this process, and sinusitis can result when bacteria from the nose get inside the sinus and multiply faster than the body can get rid of them.

Recent research has shown that many or possibly most URIs are associated with some degree of inflammation of the sinuses. While that would technically be called sinusitis, what we generally mean when we use the word is bacterial infection of the sinus cavity. The main symptom of this is increased drainage from the nose. If there is a lot of pressure inside the sinus, there can also be pain and swelling evident on the outside of the face, but this is uncommon in children. If most URIs cause at least a little bit of sinusitis, when should we consider treating it? There are some recommendations based upon recent research to keep in mind. These recommendations take into account the fact that all URIs are accompanied by increased nasal discharge.

We treat sinusitis when one of these situations apply: there is persistent nasal drainage for greater than ten days; more severe symptoms are present—for example, fever and cloudy drainage for three to four days; or substantial nasal drainage returns after first going away. As you can see, sinusitis is never anything that needs attention in the middle of the night. If you think your child has it, the matter can always wait at least until morning.

Another thing to know about sinusitis in children is that sinusitis is what we term a *clinical diagnosis*, meaning we do not need blood tests or x-rays. We sometimes do get x-rays of the sinuses in complicated situations, but they are not needed most times. In fact, they can be confusing; what they identify is inflammation in the sinuses, and since URIs nearly always inflame the sinuses to some extent, if you rely on an x-ray for deciding whether or not to use antibiotics, you will be over-treating many cases.

Sore throat is another kind of URI common in children. The reason the throat is sore is that it is inflamed, and inflamed tissue hurts, whether it is from viruses infecting the lining cells of the throat or the painful swelling that follows hitting your thumb with a hammer. The majority of sore throats are caused by respiratory viruses, and there is no specific treatment. But as nearly all parents know, another cause for a sore throat is infection with a bacteria with the scientific name of *Streptococcus pyogenes*, or *strep* for short. You read a little about strep in the last chapter, but here are some more details. I have noticed over the years that many parents have misconceptions about strep throats, and more than a few have an unreasonable fear of them, so the more information you have the better.

The strep bacteria gets passed around among children in the same way that respiratory viruses do, with touching infected hands being the most common. When it gets in the back of the throat, it multiplies like other infecting microorganisms. It is interesting that it does not always invade and cause problems. If you do throat cultures on a hundred normal children you will find a few of them harboring strep but having no symptoms. Except in unusual situations, we do not give such children antibiotic treatment, which is one reason we do not do throat cultures on children without symptoms—a positive result may be more confusing than helpful. Strep is more likely than respiratory viruses to cause the release of those fever-causing substances you read about in chapter 3, so a high temperature is common. Also common, besides the throat hurting, are headache and abdominal pain.

When you shine a light in the back of the throat of a child with a sore throat, you see much the same thing whether the cause is a virus or strep. Redness from the inflammation and enlarged tonsils are typical, the result of the body fighting off the infection. The tonsils are examples of what we call *lymph tissue*. They are regional headquarters for an important part of the immune system, the base for key infection-fighting cells. When there is an infection in the region, the lymph tissue swells as reinforcements from the immune system arrive on the scene. The battle between the body's cells and the invading germs causes casualties; the grey-white flecks you often see on the tonsils during a URI are cells killed in the struggle.

The tonsils are only part of the lymph tissue in the mouth and throat. There are also lumps called *lymph nodes* in the neck below the jaw, and these often become inflamed too. The result is the tender, "swollen glands" you can feel with your fingers. The swelling of these nodes combines with the inflamed tissue in the back of the throat to make it painful to swallow.

Most parents know the way to tell if a sore throat is strep and not a virus is to do a throat culture. This involves rubbing a cotton swab on the inflamed tissues, typically the tonsils, and then making a culture of the material on the swab in the laboratory to see if any strep bacteria are there. This process takes a day or two. To speed things along, we have the *rapid strep screen*, which is a test in which the laboratory can treat the swab with an agent that recognizes strep. It is a handy test and gives a quick answer, but it is also not as sensitive as the culture, so sometimes the rapid screen can be negative and the strep can still be identified a day later when the culture results come back.

The strep test (culture or rapid screen) is the only way to tell if a sore throat is viral or strep. You cannot tell by looking at it. It is a common misconception that really red, swollen tonsils covered with a grey discharge of dead inflammatory cells are more likely to indicate strep than ones that do not look so inflamed, but that is not so. However, there are a few things that make strep more likely. One is the child's age. For example, strep is very rare in young toddlers compared with school-age children. If the child has a runny nose and is sneezing, the sore throat is more likely to be viral. If an older child has fever, a sore throat, a headache, and belly pain, it is more likely to be strep. Being exposed to a known case of strep also makes it more likely. But none of these tendencies are solid enough to be sure—only the strep test will do that.

The distinction between strep and viral sore throats is an important one because we treat strep with antibiotics. What many parents do not know is that we do not treat the strep to make the sore throat heal more quickly—that happens on its own either way—but to prevent serious (and quite rare) complications of strep that can appear later. These are rheumatic fever, which is a heart problem; an inflammation of the kidneys called *glomerulonephritis*; and a really rare neurological problem called *chorea*. There also are complications that strep can cause around the tonsils, such as an abscess, but those take days to develop.

The reason to know these things about strep is to understand that strep throat never needs immediate treatment in the middle of the night. If your child has a red, sore throat and swollen neck glands, you can wait until the next day at least to get a strep test. It is a contentious subject even among doctors, but rigorous research has never demonstrated that early treatment makes the child get better faster. You can prevent the potential complications of strep I listed above merely by treating the infection within a few days.

Before we get to some specific case examples, you should also know a little about cough, since a cough is such a common part of a URI. It is also common with infections down further in the breathing system, such as the lungs. You will read about that in the next chapter. A cough is part of the body's natural defenses against outside invasion. We have tiny sensors in the upper airway that trigger a cough when they are stimulated. Think of them as tripwires put there to detect unwanted material and keep it from getting deep into the lungs. Not surprisingly, the area at and just below the vocal cords has a particularly dense network of cough sensors because that is where an inhaled particle, such as a bit of food or a wayward mosquito, will touch first on its way to the lung. You experience this if you drink a sip of water and a little hits the top of your voice box (*larynx*), the gateway to the lungs; the result is a powerful series of coughs. When those areas become inflamed by a URI, the cough sensors are stimulated frequently, particularly by the increased mucous the infection causes.

The main thing to understand about cough is that by itself it can mean many things. We need to evaluate it in the context of other problems the child is having, such as breathing troubles. You will read much more about those in the next chapter. Now we can look closely at our scenarios to help you decide what to do if your child develops a URI, cough, or earache.

WATCHFUL WAITING

Your two-year-old has had a cough and runny nose for a couple of days. It seems to come at random times during the day, although she does not wake up at night coughing. She also is eating well and has her normal level of activity. She has had no fever. The cough is mostly dry, but every now and then it gets wetter and she coughs up some phlegm. It is Friday evening and your family is leaving the next day for a week-long trip out of town. The cough seems worse, although your daughter is otherwise acting the same. You are worried about her getting worse during the trip and that maybe something needs to be done now for her. Does it? Should you give her a dose of an over-the-counter cough medicine?

This case is a good example of when it is most appropriate to use watchful waiting. The child does not show any signs of serious illness. The key point is that there is nothing a physician would do for this child were you to bring her to the emergency department. That is an important way to think about all these decisions: what would the doctor do? Here the doctor would simply tell you to watch for signs of worsening breathing problems, something you will learn a great deal about in the next chapter.

Many parents wonder if over-the-counter remedies, such as cough medicines and decongestants, are useful and appropriate for children like this. The American Academy of Pediatrics, among other professional societies, advises against their use. They do not help much, if at all, and they can have unpleasant side effects, such as drowsiness or behavioral changes. So assuming you will be somewhere on your trip where you could see a doctor in the highly unlikely possibility things got worse, you can safely make your trip.

WATCHFUL WAITING

Our next case features your two-year-old son, who has had a runny nose and cough for a couple of days. Now at midnight his congestion is much worse, and he has a fever of 103 degrees. He is also digging in his left ear as if it hurts. He has had several ear infections in the past and they all started the same way: a couple of days of runny nose, followed by a fever and fussiness that heralded the beginning of the ear problem. You think he probably has another one. He is irritable, but alert. What should you do?

The answer to this one should be easy and straightforward to you after what you have read earlier in the chapter. It is highly likely he does indeed have an ear infection. Many parents choose to bring children such as this to the emergency department, and I have seen many just like him in my time working there. You could certainly do that. But as you read earlier in the chapter, there is nothing wrong with giving him something for his fever and then using a strategy of watchful waiting for the rest of the night. If he is still having fever in the morning, you could take him to the doctor then.

CALL THE DOCTOR

This case also involves a cough, but this time it is in your six-year-old, who has been intermittently coughing for weeks. You have noticed it is worse at night, and particularly worse after he has been running around for a few minutes. This evening he was out playing vigorously with his friends and came back in the house with a coughing fit. The symptoms are much better now, a half-hour later, and he is now playing comfortably without being short of breath or coughing. You wonder if you should get him checked out tonight because, although you realize the cough has been going on for a considerable time, you are concerned his worse episode tonight means he needs to see a doctor now.

The way to look at this situation is to assess how he is now, after the worse coughing spell has passed, and now he is better. However, he clearly has a chronic coughing problem, and it would be good to have that evaluated, just not tonight. His brief period of worsening during the evening is a sign to take some action. It is not an emergency, or even urgent, but it is something that needs attention. So the best course of action is to call the doctor. More than likely the doctor will suggest that you arrange for the child to be seen in the next several days.

CHECKLIST AND ACTION PLANS FOR COUGHS, SNEEZES, SORE THROATS, AND EARACHES

The action plans for this chapter revolve around the key question of whether or not the problem is potentially worse than it appears, because simple URIs, sore throats, and earaches do not require prompt medical attention in the middle of the night. If your child has more symptoms than these, for example breathing problems or lethargy, then you will find appropriate action plans in later chapters. For this chapter we only have two categories to deal with.

Watchful Waiting

1. Other than perhaps being a bit fussy, your child is alert and acting normally.
2. Your child is drinking normally.
3. There are no breathing problems besides perhaps a mild cough.

Call the Doctor

1. Along with the other symptoms, your child has had a fever for over twenty-four hours.
2. Your child is not drinking well.
3. Your child is not as active and alert as he is normally.

5

BREATHING TROUBLES

A very large number of the families in the waiting rooms of America's emergency departments are there because their child has some problem with breathing. The child could be breathing too fast and hard, have trouble catching his breath, or have trouble getting air in, out, or both. Breathing troubles are often frightening to both parents and their child. Anxiety, in turn, often can make the original problem even worse. It can be a self-reinforcing cycle. In this chapter you will learn how doctors evaluate breathing problems. As with the previous chapters, after we discuss some of the general principles, we will use the specific scenarios to see how these principles are put into action.

You can think of breathing issues as falling into one of two categories. The first is trouble with the upper airway, which starts at the nose, goes on to the back of the throat, and then extends down to the area just below the larynx, or voice box. You can feel your larynx as the hard cartilage at the front of your neck, the Adam's apple. The second category is trouble down in the lung, which itself can be divided into two sorts of troubles that correspond to the two principal regions of the lung.

The first part of the lung consists of the conducting airways, the tubes that carry the air in and out. These are like the branches of an upside-down tree, beginning with the trunk as the windpipe in the neck and ending with the tiny twigs, the smallest air tubes. The business part of the lung is where gas exchange—oxygen for carbon dioxide—happens. Oxygen moves into the bloodstream from air we breathe in, and it is then distributed throughout the body. Carbon dioxide, a principal waste product of our body's burning of fuel, moves out of the body, carried by the air we exhale. The exchange of oxygen for carbon dioxide happens in tiny air sacs that sit on the ends of the smallest air tubes like clusters of grapes. Bathing the walls of the clusters are blood vessels that soak up the oxygen and dump out the carbon dioxide.

All three components—the upper airway, the lower conducting airways, and the air sacs—can be the source of breathing troubles bad enough to bring a child to the emergency department. But understanding how the lungs and airways work can help parents make practical, appropriate decisions about whether or not they should wait and see how things go, call the doctor, or bring their child to the emergency department. This chapter will help you do that.

We start with the upper airway. It has two jobs to do. The first is to let air pass by easily to the lower airways and on to the air sacs. The second is to humidify the air as it passes by, since dry air would damage the deep parts of the lung. Of these two jobs, it is the first that can lead to trouble—the free passage of air can be partially blocked. A stuffy nose blocks airflow, but a child can compensate by breathing though his mouth. Once the nasal passages join with the passage from the mouth, significant narrowing of the pipeline can cause symptoms, the severity of which matches the severity of the narrowing.

No matter what the cause of the narrowing, and there are several common ones that we will discuss, the symptoms are the same—air hunger. The muscles of the chest are powerful, and they can pull very hard against the narrowed airway to force air into the lungs.

The effect is similar to trying to suck air through a very narrow straw. The increased force of the chest muscles working hard to pull in air causes the base of the neck to suck in right above the breastbone. That is what you can see. What you can hear is a very characteristic crowing noise called *stridor*. It is the sound of air rushing rapidly through a narrowed passageway.

The most common cause of significant upper airway obstruction in children is *croup*. This is a disorder caused by inflammation of the area just below the vocal cords, called the *subglottic region*. Even though the inflammation can stretch up and down the airway, it is in the subglottic region where the symptoms happen. Why this is so is because of simple physics—that is where the upper airway of a small child is at its narrowest. The symptoms of croup come from blockage of airflow at this critical point.

The inflammation of the subglottic region makes the lining of the windpipe, or *trachea*, swell. Since the trachea is more or less round, this swelling makes the diameter of the airway smaller. Sometimes the swelling of the tissues gets so bad the size of the child's airway is narrowed to that of a small straw. What happens next is simple physics, and is analogous to what happens in cold-water pipes if they have their diameter narrowed by mineral deposits in them: flow through a tube is proportional to the fourth power of the radius of the tube. This may sound esoteric, but the principle has important practical implications for small children with croup.

Imagine an adult whose airway has a diameter of twelve millimeters. Now imagine the lining of this tube develops one millimeter of swelling all around its lining, thereby reducing its diameter to ten millimeters. If you do the calculations, this slight reduction in size reduces airflow by about half. Now consider a toddler with a five-millimeter airway that has the same one millimeter of swelling all the way around it, reducing it to three millimeters in diameter. The adult in this example loses about half the airflow, something easily compensated for by just breathing a little harder. In contrast, the toddler has his airflow reduced to only 13 percent of what it was. This reduction is very difficult to compensate for, although the child tries. His trying causes the tugging at the base of the neck and the stridor—the symptoms of croup.

There is another reason this obstruction causes trouble for a small child. The front portion of a toddler's ribcage is not yet solid bone; it is still partly cartilage. This means that, since a child's chest does not yet have the firm scaffolding of the ribs to support it, the increased effort of breathing makes the chest cave in the wrong way with each breath. These are called *retractions*. They are not specific to croup because they can happen in a child with respiratory distress from a variety of causes. The final characteristic finding of croup—a seal-like, barking cough—is from irritation of the vocal cords and the region just below them.

One of the characteristic attributes of croup is how suddenly it can cause trouble. Another is that for some reason, croup tends to be worse at night; most visits to emergency departments for croup occur between ten in the evening and four in the morning. A typical story is that parents put their child to bed with just a mild cough, only to awaken in the middle of the night to the sound of severe stridor. This is a predictable result of how the inflammation of croup happens. A child can tolerate some degree of airway narrowing. But if the croup worsens only a little bit, the resulting further reduction in airway size, though small, becomes critical. Then the symptoms suddenly worsen. What parents need to decide is what to do in the middle of the night when their child has this common condition.

There are a few other causes of upper airway obstruction besides croup that are worth knowing about. The key thing to remember is that anything that blocks airflow between the mouth and the lungs will give similar symptoms—the tugging of the chest as the child works to get air in and the characteristic sound of air rushing through the narrowed passageway.

Sometimes the narrowing happens above the place affected by croup—the soft tissues at the back of the throat. This is usually from infection. The tonsils are back there, and infected tonsils can get quite large. However, it is uncommon for even quite large tonsils to block off airflow sufficiently to cause severe symptoms. The soft tissues behind or beside the tonsils can become swollen too, but significant obstruction of breathing does not happen very often there either, although the child can have other symptoms of infection, like fever and sore throat.

Other than croup, there is one other important infectious cause of upper airway obstruction in children. It is now extremely rare, and it is a good thing that it is. In the neck the windpipe lies in front of the *esophagus*, the tube through which we swallow food into our stomachs. That means when we swallow food it must pass over the opening to the windpipe to get to the esophagus behind it. The epiglottis is a flap of tissue that covers the windpipe as we swallow so we do not get food down into our lungs. It opens as we breath in and out using a hinge mechanism much like the kind of kitchen trash can that flips open when you step on the foot pedal.

If the epiglottis, the lid of the trash can, becomes swollen it is easy to see how it could obstruct air going down into the windpipe. The condition in which this happens is called *epiglottitis*, and it can be life-threatening. Unlike croup, epiglottitis also interferes with normal swallowing because the epiglottis is so swollen it blocks the path to the esophagus too. So a child with epiglottitis not only has trouble breathing, he also has trouble swallowing. As a result he typically has drooling of his saliva. The great majority of cases of epiglottitis were caused by a bacteria with the scientific name of *Haemophilus influenza*, or HIB for short. We have had an effective vaccine against HIB for many years now, and as a result epiglottitis is fortunately quite rare, unless the child has not been vaccinated against the germ.

Breathing problems beyond the upper airway, out in the lung itself, behave differently. There are several common ones that bring children to the emergency department, and for all of them parents can understand enough about what is going on to make appropriate decisions regarding what to do—stay home and watch, call the doctor, or come to the emergency department.

Asthma is the most common breathing problem of childhood, and it is becoming more common. There are various theories about why this is so, but whatever the reason, as of this writing approximately 10 percent of all children in America have some form of asthma. The disorder varies in seriousness from mild to severe. A very large proportion of children whose parents bring them to the emergency department for breathing problems are there because of asthma. If your child has asthma, you probably already know a good deal about it. But you may not know how doctors evaluate asthma attacks; understanding how we look at it will help you make good decisions with your own child.

Asthma is a complicated condition. It represents the lung's response to things that irritate it. The main problem in asthma is that the conducting airway system gets blocked in several ways, so oxygen cannot get into the body and carbon dioxide cannot leave it. Although both are a problem in a severe asthma attack, getting the air out is usually a bigger issue than getting it in because it is easier for us to generate more force sucking in air than blowing it out.

So the hallmark of asthma is not getting the air out—called *air trapping*. Why does this happen? There are three principal reasons. For one, the smallest of airways deep in the lung, called the *bronchioles*, get even smaller because they are pinched by bands of muscle that surround them—the effect is similar to screwing down tiny hose clamps. For another, the walls of the bronchioles swell, reducing their diameter. Finally, the airways fill with excess mucous, further blocking air flow. Why do these things happen?

Both the muscle bands around the bronchioles and the mucous are there for good reasons. The lungs need a way to direct the air we breathe in to the best spots, which are those regions of the lung with the best blood flow, and that changes from minute to minute because of such things as changes in our position—lying down to standing up, for example. Those muscle bands function like the head gates of an irrigation system, opening and closing to direct air to the best places. The mucous is important because it is one of the chief defenses our lungs have against harmful or irritating things we breathe in. The mucous traps debris and steadily moves it up and out of our lungs, using a conveyer-belt system similar to the one you read about for the middle ear and sinuses.

In asthma, both of these natural systems become deranged. The muscle bands constrict when they should not, reducing air flow, and the production of mucous becomes so excessive that it plugs things up. The so-called triggers for this derangement vary from person to person, but the results are similar: air cannot move normally.

The typical symptom of asthma is wheezing. This is the sound the child makes as she tries to empty air out of her lungs. It is a high-pitched sound, easy to hear with a stethoscope against the chest, and often it can be heard even without a stethoscope. A more subtle sign is a prolongation of expiration; the child is getting the air out with each breath, but it takes her longer to do so. The child also is short of breath and typically has a frequent cough. If you have a child with asthma, you are probably familiar with all these things. You also probably have medicines at home to use when your child has an asthma attack. But how do you decide when home therapy is not doing the job and it is time to make a trip to the emergency department? We will talk about that when we get to some specific scenarios.

There is another air trapping problem that mimics an asthma attack in many ways, but is instead an infection caused by one of several viruses, the most common of which is called *respiratory syncytial virus*, or RSV for short. The condition is called *bronchiolitis*, and it most commonly happens in small infants. It is extremely common during the winter months. Babies with bronchiolitis have their smallest lung airways, the bronchioles, blocked by inflammation and mucous. Their symptoms are typically rapid breathing, cough, wheezing, and retractions, those inward movements of the lower ribs when they breathe. Their airways are already small to begin with, and the extra mucous can quickly cause blockage of airflow.

Up until now we have been discussing problems with getting air in and out of the lungs. There are also a large number of children visiting the emergency department who are there because they have breathing difficulties related to problems down in the air sacs, the place where oxygen enters the blood and carbon dioxide leaves. The most common of these disorders is *pneumonia*.

The reason children with pneumonia have breathing issues is that when the air gets down to the air sacs it finds them plugged, or even filled, with debris, usually fluid. So the air goes in and out just fine, but the air never meets the blood to exchange the oxygen for carbon dioxide. There is what we call *mismatching* of blood flow and air flow—the two never meet up as they should. There are many different kinds of pneumonia, ranging from mild (requiring no medical attention) to very severe. The very word *pneumonia* can cause fear in parents, and especially grandparents, but the great majority of children with pneumonia are only mildly to moderately ill. In children, the most common causes are infections, either from viruses or bacteria.

Children with breathing problems from pneumonia behave differently than children with croup, asthma, or bronchiolitis. Pneumonia often has a prominent cough, more so than asthma. The air goes in and out just fine, so there is not the stridor you hear in a child with croup who is breathing as though through a straw. Although sometimes children with pneumonia have wheezing, especially if they have asthma already, generally wheezing is not a significant issue. What is typical for pneumonia is rapid breathing. There is often fever, because most pneumonias are caused by infection. The oxygen content of the blood may be lower than normal, leading to bluish discoloration around the lips. Infants with pneumonia often show retractions because they are working harder to breathe; the infection makes their lungs stiffer, less limber.

In children, most pneumonias are caused by viruses, not bacteria, so we have no specific treatment for them because antibiotics do not kill viruses. For a physician examining a child with pneumonia, however, there is no way to tell the difference, so most children with pneumonia end up being treated with antibiotics. Often the doctor can diagnose pneumonia by listening to the child's chest with a stethoscope, but this is a disorder for which an x-ray is usually the way to tell what is going on in the lungs. The x-ray can also help the doctor decide what sort of pneumonia it is.

Now that you have learned about the main categories of breathing troubles—upper airway blockage, lower airway blockage, and trouble in the air sacs—it is time to see how these things show themselves when your child is sick in the middle of the night and you are trying to decide if you need to go to the emergency department.

WATCHFUL WAITING

Your six-month-old child has had a mild cough for several days. He has otherwise been normal in his activity, eating, and sleeping. Now you notice he has a fever of 101 degrees. You know that the fever by itself is not a reason to do anything other than perhaps give him medicine for it. But when you look at him lying on his back, it seems he is breathing faster than normal. You read somewhere that breathing rate is important, and you time it with your watch; he is taking about forty breaths each minute. His breathing is not labored in any way—it just is a bit fast. What should you do?

This is a good opportunity to talk about what is a normal breathing rate for a child and how to measure it. Breathing rate varies with age, and it even varies minute to minute depending upon what the person is doing. So it is important to look at trends and averages; you should not make any decisions from just one measurement, particularly in very small children. Respiratory rate is calculated as the number of breaths in a minute. It is hard to count out an entire minute, so an easy way is to count the number of breaths in fifteen seconds and then multiply by four. Sometimes it can be hard to see the breaths, so lift your child's shirt up to see better. Do it several times and average the result.

An infant normally takes anywhere from thirty to forty breaths per minute, with brief periods of time when the rate can normally be as high as sixty. Toddlers and preschoolers have lower rates, normally about twenty to thirty. By the time a child is school age, he has a rate near to that of an adult—fourteen to twenty or so. Understand that these are broad ranges, steadily decreasing from the relatively rapid and variable rate of an infant to the slow, steady rate of an older child or adult.

There are several things that increase a child's respiratory rate, particularly that of an infant or toddler. Activity is one, agitation and irritability are others. Fever also raises respiratory rate, so if your child has a high temperature and is breathing faster, this does not necessarily mean there is anything wrong with his airway or lungs.

Knowing all this, what is the best course of action for the parent of the child described above? He has had what sounds like a URI, a cold, for several days. Now his breathing rate is a bit increased for his age. But he also has a fever, and that typically raises the rate. So one thing to do is to give the child something for his high temperature and then see what his breathing rate is after the fever comes down.

The most important thing to understand is that breathing rate needs to be considered not in isolation, but in relation to other things the child is doing. The most important concept, and one doctors use all the time in evaluating children with breathing problems, is what we term *work of breathing*. The concept is to try to evaluate objectively what a small child cannot describe to you. An older child or adult can describe how they feel. For example, they can tell you if they feel short of breath or have difficulty catching their breath, both of which are subjective feelings, not things we can measure.

Babies and small children cannot tell us how they are feeling; we have to figure it out by looking at them. Experienced examiners, and that can certainly include parents, learn how to do this. What we call work of breathing plays an important role in the assessment. The first step is to measure respiratory rate. Next, we look at a couple of things that tell us if the child is working harder at getting air in and out. An important sign in children under six months or so, and sometimes older, are those retractions. You read a little about them earlier, but we should discuss their cause in a bit more detail.

The ribcage surrounds the lungs, forming a stiff container that helps hold the lungs open. The cage has a set of joints at the point where the front of the ribs join the breastbone. These joints are made of cartilage, which is firm but softer than bone. You can feel the difference if you touch your nose. The bone at the bridge of you nose is hard, the cartilage at the tip is not. This set of ribcage hinges is important because the chest cavity needs to expand and contract as we breathe in and out. The bars of the cage, the rib bones, also can move apart from one another as we breathe, giving more space for the lung to expand.

If you feel the front of a six-month-old child's chest, you can detect the ribs, but what you are feeling is not bone, but cartilage. A child's ribs do not become fully bone up to the point where they meet the joints at the breastbone until several years of age. This means an infant or young toddler does not have a completely firm cage for his lungs, and it has important consequences when we decide if a child has increased work of breathing.

When a small child is working harder than normal to breathe, she is using her chest muscles to generate more force with each breath. When that happens, her chest cage tends to sink in, rather than expand out, with each breath. This shows itself by the breastbone sinking rather than rising and the lowest ribs moving inward rather than outward. A somewhat older child, one whose ribcage is more completely formed, may have inward movement at the base of the neck above the breastbone. Retractions are a key indicator that a child is having increased work of breathing.

Now let us return to the six-month-old with the somewhat rapid breathing and the fever. If this were your child, what you should do is first give him something to bring down his fever. Even if that does not work, you can still make a good assessment of the situation. Just look at him carefully. Does he seem alert? Or does he have a look in his eyes that suggests he is devoting his mind to breathing rather than looking at you? If he is concentrating on breathing rather than you, it is a good sign that his work of breathing is increased. Does he have any retractions of his breastbone or under his lower ribs? If he does, then his work of breathing is definitely increased.

This particular child is breathing faster than normal, but he has no evidence of increased work of breathing—no retractions. He has a fever, but as you learned in the last chapter, that does not necessarily mean you need to do anything more than give him acetaminophen or ibuprofen. He is also alert. The bottom line is that, if this were your child, you could use watchful waiting and observe him to see how things go.

CALL THE DOCTOR

Your three-year-old daughter has been coughing all day. The cough is dry, without any phlegm, and as the evening progresses it sounds more and more like a barking seal. She is eating and drinking normally and has no fever. In between her coughing spells she is breathing normally. What should you do?

This child has typical croup. The barking cough gives it away. The cough is irritating, but what you are looking for here is evidence that airway obstruction is happening. To do this you use your eyes and your ears. You look to see if she has any retractions, and you listen to hear if she has any sound of stridor, that sound of air rushing through a narrowed passageway. This particular child has only the barking cough right now.

If you are an old hand at croup, perhaps having seen it before in your other children, you certainly could watch and see what happens. You could try one of the traditional remedies for croup, which is to soothe the child's inflamed airway with warm, moist air. The standard way to do this is to close the bathroom door and run a very hot shower for several minutes, filling the air with steam. Then turn off the shower and sit with the child in the bathroom, breathing the moist air. An even older remedy is to use cold air, done by taking the child outside into the cold night air. This is often possible because croup is more common in the colder months of the year. Opinions vary over the benefits of these remedies, but there is no harm in giving them a try. What would make you consider bringing your child to the emergency department?

The key thing to look for is what doctors call *stridor at rest*. A typical child with croup can have intermittent mild stridor. It appears when the child is agitated and breathing faster, then it disappears when the child is calm. If your child is calm and still has stridor, then you should bring him in to be seen. We have medications that will help treat the airway inflammation and swelling and keep things from getting worse.

There are two common medicines for croup we use in the emergency department. Both work by decreasing the swelling of the airway. The first of these is called *epinephrine*. It works by shrinking swollen tissues. We give it by making it into a mist and having the child breathe it in, and it works very quickly, usually within minutes. It does not last very long, however, perhaps an hour or so, which is why if your child receives inhaled epinephrine, the doctor will generally keep him there for at least another hour to see if the swelling comes back and the stridor returns. The second medicine we use for croup is a *steroid*, either taken by mouth, inhaled as a mist, or given as a shot in the muscle. Steroids are very effective in treating croup inflammation, but they do not work right away. They take several hours to kick in, but then they work to keep the inflammation under control for many hours afterward.

GO TO THE EMERGENCY DEPARTMENT

Your six-year-old son has had a chronic cough for months. It is especially worse after energetic playing. It has always passed within an hour at most. Tonight, though, he seems to be having more trouble. After a summer evening of vigorous running around, he has to sit down to catch his breath. Every so often he seems to heave his chest up higher to get a good breath. When you ask him how he feels, he has to pause and take several short breaths before he can finish each sentence in his answer. What should you do with him?

This child is having an asthma attack. There are a couple of things that tell you this. He has been coughing for several months; often asthma gives symptoms of chronic cough. Children with asthma also typically have triggers that bring on an attack, and exercise is a common one. This child as well demonstrates a common finding with asthma, one that doctors often use in assessing how much trouble an older child is having getting air out of his lungs: we ask the child to speak a string of words, such as counting to ten. A child who is significantly short of breath will not be able to speak more than a few words without stopping to take a breath. The child in this scenario has to pause and take several short breaths before he can finish each sentence in his answer, indicating that he is having real problems.

If this were your child, what should you do? If the child has never had breathing problems like this before, then it is best to take him to the emergency department. If the child has had problems like this in the past, you may already have asthma medicine, such as albuterol, at home. If this is the case, you can give him a breathing treatment and see how he does. If he is no better in fifteen to thirty minutes, you can give him another one. If he still is not significantly better, then you should bring him to the emergency department. The doctors there will repeat the albuterol and also give him other treatments, such as oxygen and steroids.

The key point is that his breathing troubles may well get worse, and after you have given him a couple of albuterol treatments, there is nothing else you can do at home to improve things. So watchful waiting, or even calling the doctor, is not the best option. If he does not significantly improve in the emergency department, he may need to be admitted to the hospital.

CALL 911

This scenario casts you forward a year. In the previous scenario you took your son to the emergency department, he received various breathing treatments, and he got better. They sent him home with some prescriptions for these same medicines, and you took him to his doctor the following week. His doctor said he had asthma and that he should continue to take several of the medicines. A few weeks after that the doctor modified his program a bit, changing him to an inhaled medicine he has taken twice each day since. Overall he has done quite well during the past year. He had a few times when he seemed to breathe harder and have a cough, but taking a bit more of one of the inhaled medicines took care of the problem.

Now he suddenly is having much worse troubles. He seemed fine at dinnertime, except maybe for an occasional cough. Now you awaken in the middle of the night to hear him coughing from down the hall. When you go to his room you find him sitting bolt upright in bed. He can barely speak at all, and with each breath his shoulders rise a couple of inches. You give him a breathing treatment with one of the medications, as your doctor has told you to do in situations like this, and he gets a little better. Fifteen minutes later you give another treatment, but he seems about the same. What should you do? It certainly looks as if he needs more and stronger treatments than you can give at home. Should you call somebody, perhaps the nurse help line your doctor's office uses at night?

What we are looking at in this scenario is a true emergency because children in this situation can quickly progress to not being able to move much air in and out of the lung at all. If this child were your child you should not take him to the emergency department in your car—you should call 911 for help. While waiting for the ambulance to get there you could give him more albuterol, but you should make the call first. The paramedics will bring with them additional treatments they can get started right away, particularly oxygen.

CHECKLIST AND ACTION PLANS FOR BREATHING TROUBLES

The most important concept to keep in mind is that the underlying reason for the breathing problem—whether upper airway obstruction, obstruction in the small airways, or abnormalities in the small air sacs—does not matter as much as how the child looks, how much distress she is in. With that in mind, here is a checklist with some general principles to help you decide what to do. As with the last chapter, a good way to use the list is to move your action plan up to the next level if you are unsure of what you are seeing.

Watchful Waiting

1. Your child's breathing rate is normal for age or only a little elevated (less than fifty for an infant, forty for a toddler, thirty for an older child).
2. There are no retractions.
3. Your child is alert and able to drink fluids normally.

Call the Doctor

1. Your child's breathing rate is faster than fifty for an infant, forty for a toddler, or thirty for an older child.
2. There are minimal retractions, ones that you need to look closely to notice.
3. Your child is alert and drinking fluids well.
4. There may be some stridor with agitation, but there is no stridor at rest.

Take Your Child to the Emergency Department

1. Your child's breathing rate is much faster than fifty for an infant, forty for a toddler, or thirty for an older child.
2. There are more severe retractions, ones that are obvious at a glance.
3. There is stridor at rest.
4. Your child has wheezing that does not improve significantly after two albuterol treatments (if you have such medications at home).

Call 9 1 1

1. Your child is barely able to move air in and out.
2. Your child is poorly responsive.
3. Your child's color is poor, such as a bluish color around the face.

6

DIGESTIVE AND ABDOMINAL PROBLEMS

Belly aches, vomiting, and diarrhea—issues of the digestive system—are common childhood problems. They are so common no child gets through childhood without experiencing them, and a fair number of the children in any emergency department waiting room will be there because of them. These problems can be especially vexing to parents because, unlike viral URIs, digestive problems run the gamut from trivial to very serious, and most parents are well aware of this. They know these problems often require no particular therapy, but they also know one or two of them could potentially require emergency surgery. It is worry about the latter category that brings a family to the emergency department.

As with all the topics in this book, my goal in this chapter is not to replace a doctor's judgment with your own. But any parent can understand the principles doctors use to decide where on the severity spectrum their child's complaints are. More than that, any parent can put these principles into practice, perhaps saving you and your child a late-night trip to the emergency department.

Before we get into specific problems, it is very helpful to learn some useful facts about the digestive system—what its job is, and the kinds of things that can go wrong. If you understand that, you are in a good position to understand where symptoms of digestive problems come from.

The digestive system starts in the mouth and extends all the way to the rectum. Its job, of course, is to deal with everything we eat and drink. It sorts through all this material and decides what to do with it. It has several choices. They range from absorbing the material into the body unchanged, breaking down the material—digesting it—and then absorbing it, or simply allowing what we have swallowed to pass through unchanged.

There is one aspect of the digestive system that is interesting to think about for a moment because it is a useful notion. Although we think of the digestive system as being inside us, it really is not—it is a continuation of the outside world. It is a long tunnel, a cave, that opens to the environment on both ends. This is an important concept because many digestive problems result from the body's need to control things that are happening within the cave. The body needs to make sure what belongs in the cave stays there. For example, the cave is full of bacteria, and there is always a danger of these germs breaking out of the cave's interior and causing troubles either in the immediate area or in the rest of the body.

Although in general the microscopic world of the digestive system is teeming with germs, this varies by location. Beginning at the top, the mouth is full of germs. In fact, it is so germ-laden that a deep bite from a human is more likely to cause serious infection than one from a dog. The path from the mouth to the stomach leads down the *esophagus*, the swallowing tube. The esophagus is made of muscle that squeezes food onward into the cave. The stomach is not free of germs, but because of the acid there, their numbers are much smaller. The portion of the cave below the stomach is the small intestine, which is divided into several segments. The further down you go, the higher the germ concentration. By the time you reach the large intestine, or *colon*, the germ concentrations are enormous—many billions of them in a teaspoon of intestinal contents.

Why are all those germs there, and how did they get there? The simple answer is they are there because there is nothing to prevent it. The inside of the body is sterile, germ-free. But the cave-tunnel of the digestive system is not really inside the body; it is a twisting pathway through the body. We swallow bacteria all the time because they are everywhere in the world, on every surface, and on much of what we put in our mouth. Once we swallow them, they find themselves in a nutrient feast from all of the partially digested food around them. Safe from the cold, cruel world outside the cave, and flush with all the food, they flourish and multiply.

The germs in the digestive system are part of a complicated ecosystem, an entire universe contained within our digestive cave. Among the citizens of that universe there are good germs and bad germs. The great majority are good germs, in the sense that they cause us no problems. They live out their lives peacefully, content to take what they need from the food stream passing by.

Some germs are even useful to us. For example, they provide us with vitamin K, a vitamin that is not in our food and that we cannot make ourselves. Vitamin K is key to proper blood clotting. It is so important that we routinely give it as an injection to babies when they are born because babies do not yet have any bacteria in their intestines to make it for them. Within a few days a baby's intestines begin getting populated with vitamin K–producing bacteria, and they are soon adequately supplied with it by friendly germs. If we did not give them injected vitamin K, they would be at risk for bleeding problems until they acquired their own stock of bacteria.

Mixed in with the great mass of friendly bacteria are some that are potentially quite hostile if given the chance. The opportunity they are looking for is a breakdown in the defense mechanisms the body uses to contain all the bacteria in the cave. While they wait, they are competing with all the innocent bacteria for food. In fact, the enormous mass of friendly bacteria helps out our natural defenses by keeping the hostile ones in check by taking most of the food.

This concept has practical implications worth knowing about for parents. The most common of these is the effect of antibiotic therapy. If your child has an infection, perhaps an ear infection, for which a doctor prescribes antibiotics, the medicine not only treats the ear infection; the antibiotics also cause major changes in the microbial universe in the intestines. The medicine causes a huge die-off of the benign, friendly bacteria because nearly all of them are what we term *sensitive* to the effects of the drug. Some of the potentially hostile bacteria, however, are resistant to the effects of the antibiotic. So they multiply quickly, seizing the opportunity to get a larger portion of the food supply. The result is that a larger proportion of the intestinal bacteria are potentially harmful.

The antibiotics do not kill off all of the friendly bacteria, and as soon as the antibiotics are not there, the good bacteria quickly rebound and repopulate the intestine. There are also several foods that contain live, friendly bacteria, such as acidophilus, and you can give your child foods like these to speed up the process of repopulation. Meanwhile, though, there can be problems. The most common one is diarrhea, something most parents have seen. Not surprisingly, the antibiotics more likely to cause diarrhea are the ones that kill the largest number of friendly bacteria. The effect of antibiotics on the intestinal ecosystem is one reason we should be careful in using them. They are important and generally safe medicines, but we should only use them in situations where they are clearly indicated.

Before we get to specific digestive problems, there is another thing about the body it is useful for parents to know: how digestion actually happens. This is because things that interfere with the normal digestive process are common causes of abdominal complaints.

When we drink water, we just absorb it into our body, unaltered in any fashion. For everything else, however, the digestive system has to process what we eat or drink in some way. For some substances, like simple sugars and fats, a specific transporter exists on the lining cells of the intestines to bring those into the body without further processing needed. But for most of what we eat, some breakdown of the food into its component parts has to happen in the intestine before we can absorb it. That is what digestion is.

Digestion starts in the mouth. Saliva contains substances called *enzymes* that begin the process by breaking down starchy food like bread, pasta, and potatoes. This only begins the digestive process, since much further modification of each mouthful continues after we swallow it.

Next comes the stomach, where more enzymes go to work. Now the enzyme mix includes those that break down protein, such as meat. Stomach acid also helps the process along. Another important aspect is the churning and mixing action of the stomach when it is filled with food. You can feel that at work after a large meal. The stomach makes a uniform mash of everything, then releases the mixture into the small intestine. It does this in a controlled, steady fashion by means of a valve at the stomach outlet because dumping all the stomach contents into the intestine at once, as happens in some abnormal situations, overloads the system and causes quite unpleasant symptoms.

As the food stream passes through the upper small intestine, two important digestive organs join in the process, the liver and the pancreas. The liver makes bile, which is vital to digesting fats, and the pancreas makes several key additional enzymes. Both have small tubes leading from them to the small intestine, and through which they spray the now partially digested mixture with their digestive aids.

By the time the food has reached the middle portion of the small intestine, digestion is well along and special transporter systems lining the intestine are moving the nutrients into the body. There are separate systems for fats, sugars (which are the building blocks of all carbohydrates, or "carbs") and proteins, such as meat.

The food next exits the small intestine into the large intestine, or *colon*. By now there is no useful nutrient material left—it is all absorbed. What remains is a slurry of fiber in water. The colon absorbs the excess water but does nothing to the fiber because humans, unlike animals that graze, do not have the cellular equipment to digest plant fibers in foods such as celery. These foods may contain other useful nutrients, like vitamins, but most of it cannot be digested. The fiber is important, though, because it gives the entire digestive stream bulk and helps keep moving it along. If the fiber is not there, the result, as most parents know, is constipation.

One last key point about digestion is how the food stream actually moves along, what makes it go. After all, it must be an active process—it will not move itself. The way it moves is by a process with the technical term of *peristalsis*. This is an active, muscular activity, using the muscles that surround the intestinal cave. These muscles contract in steady, coordinated waves that squeeze the intestinal contents along. The process is similar to what happens when you squeeze a half-empty toothpaste tube with your fingers to get the toothpaste in the bottom out onto your toothbrush. Normal peristalsis is important to understand because many intestinal symptoms that bring children to the emergency department are the result of the rhythmic squeezing process not working as it should. Now that you know something about the process, it is time to apply these principles to the scenarios.

WATCHFUL WAITING

Your eight-year-old son has been complaining off and on for several days that his stomach hurts. He is otherwise acting normally and has had a good appetite. You have not noticed anything associated with the pain; it seems to come and go more or less randomly. Now it is evening and he is complaining about it again, although he ate his dinner. He does not seem sick in any other way, but you had a cousin whose child once became very sick with appendicitis, and you know that starts with abdominal pain. What should you do? Does your son need to see the doctor tonight to make sure he does not have appendicitis?

This case offers us a good opportunity to talk about what questions a doctor asks to define abdominal pain. Typical questions include the following. How long has the child complained of the pain? Does it come and go or is it present all the time? Is it associated with any particular activity? Is it related to meals in any way? Are there other symptoms that go with it, such as nausea, vomiting, or diarrhea? Does the child have a fever? Is he eating and drinking normally? What is his stooling pattern? These questions help pinpoint where abdominal pain is coming from.

Abdominal pain differs from other kinds of pain, such as that from a cut in the skin, in important ways. To do their job the intestines need to be able to stretch their elastic walls quite substantially, enlarging the diameter of the cave to several times the resting state. But there is a limit to how much the tube can stretch. When that limit is reached, the pain sensing mechanism of the intestines is extremely sensitive to further stretching. What often makes the diameter suddenly bigger is gas. As all of us have experienced, gas pains are suddenly uncomfortable but are poorly localized to a specific spot. That is, if you ask someone with gas pains to point with their finger to the exact spot where it hurts, they cannot; they typically rub the general area of their abdomen.

A certain amount of gas in the intestines is normal. It gets there from air we swallow and from digestion of the foods we eat, as well as from the activities of some bacteria. But too much gas is a common cause of abdominal pain.

Abdominal pain is often what we call *crampy*. That means it comes and goes in waves. There is a minute or two of quite strong pain, followed by several minutes of little or no pain. The cramps are the result of how the intestines work, how those peristaltic muscles squeeze. The contractions normally occur every few minutes, and each one propels the intestinal contents forward. A cramp comes when a wave of muscle contraction hits a region not ready to continue the wave, such as a portion of the intestine already overfilled with gas or fluid. When that happens, the segment gets overstretched, stimulating those sensitive stretch receptors. The result is—ouch! Crampy pain can also occur if the peristaltic waves are coming faster and more vigorously than normal, as when the intestinal contents are moving along unusually quickly. That is why diarrhea is often accompanied by abdominal cramps.

Constipation, particularly chronic constipation, can cause abdominal pain in children by the same mechanism. If the large intestine, particularly the part approaching the rectum, is full of hard stool, the peristaltic waves are bumping up against an area that gets intermittently stretched. A child with pain from constipation will often have the pain come and go. Constipation pain is typically not acute, rather coming on over days. A key question to ask in this situation, of course, is if the child has had a normal stooling pattern or if his stools have been infrequent and hard in character.

Not all abdominal pain is of the crampy variety. Sometimes it is more constant, as well as being more localized. Although the stomach lining has the ability to tolerate acid in ways that other parts of the digestive system cannot, excess acid can irritate the walls of the stomach. One area that does not tolerate acid well is the lower esophagus. There is a valve at the spot where the esophagus meets the stomach that functions to keep the acid-laden stomach contents from backing up. When that safeguard malfunctions, a situation called *gastro-esophageal reflux*, the stomach contents irritate the lower esophagus, and that hurts. This kind of pain is characteristic.

It is constant, noncrampy, often associated with meals, and localized to a spot in the upper abdomen that is just below the breastbone.

One final thing to remember about abdominal pain is that it may not necessarily be coming from the digestive system at all. The abdomen is surrounded by several layers of powerful muscles. These muscles can be bruised or strained, and the result is pain over the abdomen. This variety of pain will typically be quite localized, and often the area that hurts is also tender when you touch it. Also, the kidneys lie behind the intestines, outside the abdominal cavity proper. In adults, pain from kidney problems, such as from a urinary tract infection, usually localizes to the flank, over the kidneys. In children, however, kidney problems not uncommonly cause a more diffuse pain widely distributed over the belly.

Getting back to the case in this scenario, recall that the child has been complaining of the pain for several days at least. He is otherwise acting normally and he has a good appetite. His mother has not noticed anything associated with the pain, and it seems to come and go randomly. He has not been vomiting, has no diarrhea, and he has not had fever. Now his pain is back in the evening, although he ate his dinner normally. He does not seem sick in any other way.

One thing we would really like to know about this child is his stooling pattern, because this sort of pain is typical of chronic constipation. His mother, though, is worried about appendicitis. As you will read later in the chapter, the chances of this child having appendicitis are essentially zero. In spite of this, should his parent bring him to the emergency department for evaluation of other possibilities?

The answer for this case is that watchful waiting is the best way to handle the situation. The child has had several days or more of this pain and it has not gotten any worse—the pain has simply been persistent. If the pain continues to bother him, his parent certainly could call the doctor for advice. If the child has not had a regular stooling pattern, it would be reasonable for his parent to give him a mild laxative, such as prune juice. Often a child with chronic constipation does not have much fiber or enough water in his diet, so that is another intervention that could help.

CALL THE DOCTOR

Your three-month-old daughter has been having watery stools every one or two hours for the past day. She has also vomited up her feedings a few times and seems to be feeding less vigorously than usual. She also seems a bit listless. It is now Friday evening and you are concerned she might be getting dehydrated because you have heard that infants can become dehydrated quite fast. You have also heard there is a blood test that can tell if that is happening. You wonder if you should take your daughter to the emergency department in order to get an evaluation, including blood tests. Should you?

This case can teach some useful things about vomiting and diarrhea. The child is three months old and has had both these problems for a day. She has also been listless and has not been feeding well. But before we can discuss the details of this case, we need to define our terms better. What does a doctor mean by the word *diarrhea* when considering a child of this age? After all, normal stooling pattern does change with age; infants have many more stools than older children. Individual children of the same age also have different bowel habits, so what is normal for one child may be abnormal for another.

Diarrhea is both an increase in stool frequency and a change in the character of the stools from solid or soft to runny. The stools may be so runny that they look more like dirty water than stool. What causes this? The root of the problem is usually inflammation of the lining cells of the intestines. For three-month-olds, the most common reason for the inflammation is infection from a virus, an infection called *gastroenteritis*—the "stomach flu." The medical term makes sense because the stomach, the *gastro* part of the term, is often inflamed as well as the intestines, the *entero* part of the term.

You read earlier that the upper parts of the small intestine are lined with an array of specialized absorbing cells whose job is to transport nutrients into the bloodstream. They cannot transport complex foodstuffs like meat and potatoes; these must first be broken down by the digestive enzymes into the simple building blocks that comprise them, such as sugars and protein components. The lining cells absorb this material and place it into a special part of the blood circulation that carries it all to the liver, where further processing happens. Fats are handled a little differently, but the principle of breaking down complex materials to simple ones for absorption is the same.

Inflammation injures these lining cells so they cannot do their job as well. What happens next is that some of the digested food, instead of being absorbed, continues to pass down the intestine. This material, for reasons of simple chemistry, draws water along with it, so the stools are runny. The inflammation also affects the nerves surrounding the intestines, speeding up peristalsis, and often causing crampy pain. The result is frequent, runny stools because the volume of material moving through the intestine is greater than normal. This is often (but not always) accompanied by pain.

The viruses that commonly cause this are all around us and are easily passed from child to child, especially if they are too young to wash their hands and are sharing with other children cookies, toys, and other things they put in their mouths. We have no specific treatment for viral gastroenteritis, but fortunately infections from these common viruses get cleared from the child's system within a few days. Some cause more severe symptoms than others. One in particular, called *rotavirus*, tends to do this. We now have a vaccine for rotavirus, although the illness is still common. As the infection clears, the lining cells of the intestine quickly recover, and the symptoms resolve.

There are more severe infections that cause diarrhea that are not from viruses. Several species of bacteria can do this. Their names are esoteric to non-physicians: *Campylobacter*, *Yersinia*, *Salmonella*, *Shigella*, and *E. coli*. There are also several microscopic parasites—*giardia*, *cryptosporidium*, and a few others—that can give these symptoms. These non-viral invaders tend to cause more severe symptoms and may be accompanied by high fever and blood in the stool. The fever comes from the germs' ability to stimulate the substances you read about in chapter 3; the blood is the result of more severe inflammation of the intestinal lining. Some of these infections need specific treatment.

Most of the time we cannot determine what the infecting germ is. We have no test for diarrhea-causing viruses other than rotavirus. For that one we can do a rapid test on the stool looking for it, although we have no treatment that will kill the virus. For the other germs, the bacterial and parasitic ones that cause more severe symptoms, we can send a sample of stool to the microbiology laboratory and see if any of them are present.

The child in this scenario also has vomiting—where does that come from? Vomiting is a fascinating reflex in the way it demonstrates the close link between the brain and the digestive system. The act of vomiting is a complicated and highly coordinated series of events. The brain starts the process by sending a signal to the nerves around the stomach. The stomach muscles then forcefully contract while the muscles around the valve at the entry to the stomach relax, propelling whatever is in the stomach out the mouth. At the same time the muscles around the upper airway, at the level of the vocal cords, squeeze the airway shut so that none of the material gets into the airway, an important reflex to protect our lungs.

For gastroenteritis, the signal to vomit typically is caused by the same inflammation of the digestive lining. As you will discover when we discuss appendicitis, another trigger for vomiting is when peristalsis slows down, backing up the digestive stream because very little is moving forward. The brain itself also sometimes sends a signal to vomit without any input from the digestive system at all. Most of us have experienced this phenomenon, or at least nausea, which is a precursor to vomiting, when we have met terrible smells or seen particularly distressing sights.

Now once more back to the scenario. This child has had diarrhea and is now listless. She is also feeding poorly. She has no fever and there is no blood in her stool. Her mother is worried about dehydration. It is a legitimate concern because diarrhea is the most common cause of dehydration in very small children. More than that, small infants, relative to older children and adults, become dehydrated much more easily because they have higher fluid needs. To stay hydrated, an infant weighing ten pounds needs to take in on average about an ounce and a half of fluid every two hours. An older child or adult needs much less than that. So you can see how an infant who is losing substantial amounts of water in her stool, and who is not drinking well, can become significantly dehydrated over the course of a day.

This child is listless, which is a symptom of dehydration, and is not drinking well. Her underlying illness is most certainly viral gastroenteritis, something that will pass on its own and for which we have no specific treatment anyway. The most important thing in this case is to keep her hydrated.

In this scenario, the answer is to call the doctor for advice. This is because although the child is somewhat listless, she still is alert and interactive. The doctor would ask the mother some important questions before advising what to do next. One key question is if the child is making urine. The body is excellent at holding on to fluids as much as possible, so it responds to dehydration by reducing the amount of urine. Unfortunately it can be hard to tell about urine output if a child is having watery diarrhea because the urine is often mixed with the stool. There are other clues. A dehydrated infant will make fewer tears when she cries, and her tongue and the inside of her mouth will feel dry to the touch. More severe cases cause the eyes and the soft spot on the skull to become sunken and the skin to feel doughy when you pinch it. This child has not progressed to that extent.

What the doctor is deciding from the answers to these questions is simple arithmetic: is the child taking in sufficient fluid to match the amount that is going out, plus the baseline requirement of an ounce and a half every two hours? If that is the case, then the child will not become dehydrated. There are a few things this child's parent could do to increase her drinking. One is to offer more-frequent fluids in smaller amounts, especially if the vomiting is more of a problem than the diarrhea, because a full stomach tends to worsen the vomiting.

In this case, after talking to this child's parent, the doctor decided the child did not need to be seen in the emergency department because she was still wetting her diapers and crying with tears. In spite of being a bit listless and not herself, she was still alert and interactive. He did suggest offering more-frequent fluids. The specific fluid that is best in this situation remains a matter of debate. For many years doctors routinely suggested switching from formula or breast milk to an over-the-counter electrolyte solution (Pedialyte, many others) at least for a day or so until the symptoms improved. Now some doctors suggest continuing the usual feeding. Either way, this case is one in which you do not need to take the child to the emergency department in the middle of the night, but unless you are experienced in handling this type of scenario, it would be best to call for some advice because the situation is moderately complicated.

GO TO THE EMERGENCY DEPARTMENT

This time it is a four-week-old baby who is sick. Like the infant in the preceding scenario, he has been vomiting. But what he has spit up has not just been his last feeding; the material he has vomited is thin and greenish-yellow colored. He also vomits between his attempts to feed, even when there is little to nothing in his stomach. When his vomiting started he kept trying to feed, but over the past several hours he has fed progressively less and less. Another difference from the previous scenario is that, compared with the first child, this one became sicker much faster. Twelve hours ago he was fine; now he is listless. His belly also seems a little puffed out and swollen. If this were your baby, what should you do? Should his parent watch and see how he does, maybe with more-frequent and smaller feedings?

This case illustrates some important points doctors consider in evaluating the situation. The bottom line is that this child is just plain sicker than the previous one. For one thing, he is quite listless and apathetic. He is not looking around as normal or mildly ill babies do. For another, he is younger, only a small infant. Like parents, doctors are more likely to be concerned about very small children because they are more fragile. Their ability to tolerate illness of any sort is not as robust as that of a child even a few months older. As a demonstration of that, this child became ill much faster than the previous child.

Another key point is the frequency of his vomiting. The previous child had occasional vomiting; she was not feeding as well as she usually did, but she was keeping down some fluids. The child in this scenario is vomiting up absolutely everything. So he is almost certain to be at least moderately dehydrated, since he has been doing this for twelve hours.

The nature of this child's vomiting is also different. A child with ordinary gastroenteritis typically vomits up what he eats. This child is vomiting up something else besides; he is vomiting greenish-yellow liquid. What does that mean? It means one of two things, both caused by failure of the stomach or intestinal contents to move downstream as they should. The unusual color of the fluid is from bile. Recall from what you read about normal digestion that the liver and pancreas spray the intestinal contents with substances that help digest food. The liver's contribution is bile, which has a distinctive color. The bile comes in below the stomach and moves along with the digestive stream. If the stream is not moving, the bile backs up into the stomach.

One possibility for poor movement of the digestive stream is what we call an *ileus*. This is a severe slowdown or complete cessation of peristalsis—nothing moves if the intestinal muscles do not rhythmically squeeze as they should. It is the opposite of what happens in most cases of diarrhea. The other possibility is that there is a blockage, an obstruction in the intestines. Either way, this is a serious situation. So no matter what the hour, the parents of this child should bring him to the emergency department. Once they get there, what can they expect to happen? What will the doctor do to decide what the problem is and what to do about it?

Once the doctor hears the story, she may be able to get important clues from her examination of the child. When you listen to a normal child's abdomen you can hear the sounds of peristalsis, the gurgling and rumbling all of us feel from time to time as digestion does its work. A child with an ileus will have a very quiet abdomen because peristalsis is decreased or stopped. If there is an obstruction, peristalsis continues, at least for a while, but it sounds unusually different through a stethoscope. This distinction is more difficult to tell in an infant, but the doctor may still get some hints.

While she does her evaluation, the doctor may well also start an IV, placing a small plastic tube in a hand or foot vein, to give the baby some needed fluids because this child is dehydrated from all the vomiting and inability to eat. The doctor will also probably get some blood tests. These will help her decide how dehydrated the child is, as well as give her some information about potential causes of the vomiting. The doctor will also do an examination of the child's abdomen. What she will be feeling for is some sort of lump that may be the cause of the obstruction.

One possibility is called *pyloric stenosis*. This is an enlargement of the *pylorus*, the valve at the bottom of the stomach where it joins the small intestine. The job of the pylorus is to regulate the flow of food from the large reservoir of the stomach into the intestine, making sure the food does not get dumped through all at once. For unclear reasons infants, especially boys, can experience an overgrowth of the pylorus that restricts the valve opening. The result is obstruction. It is cured by a simple operation.

Another consideration is an obstruction further down the intestine, of which there are many possibilities. Many of these are things a baby is born with, but they often do not cause obstruction symptoms right away. They also require surgery to fix, although the operations are not as simple as the one for pyloric stenosis.

This infant will probably need imaging studies to identify what is going on. Depending upon the specifics, this could mean an *ultrasound study*, which uses sound waves. This type of study will be quite good at identifying many of the possibilities of this case, particularly pyloric stenosis. Another study that may be needed is a *computed tomography* (CT) scan. This test uses x-rays coupled with what is called *contrast material*, which is placed in the stomach. The contrast helps the doctor see where the obstruction is. This particular case is one of what is called a *malrotation*, a twisting of the intestines. Like nearly all the possibilities the doctor considered for this child, it requires surgery to fix.

GO TO THE EMERGENCY DEPARTMENT

This six-year-old girl was well until yesterday morning, when she complained to her mother of vague belly pain. She went to school, but when she came home she said she felt worse. She tried to eat a little dinner, but she vomited it all up an hour later. Then she went to bed. When her mother went in to check on her, the child felt warm and in fact did have a temperature of 102 degrees. Her pain was worse. It had also changed in quality; at first it was dull and vague, now it was sharper and worse when she moved. By midnight she had not slept at all, still had a fever, and her sharp pain had worsened to the point that it hurt to move at all. The pain was mostly in the lower-right side of her abdomen.

To summarize this scenario, it is of a child with progressive abdominal pain and fever, plus some vomiting and loss of appetite. The pain was initially vague and diffuse across her abdomen, but then progressed to a sharp pain localized to the right lower part of the abdomen. By that time it hurt her to move her belly. This is a classic story for *appendicitis*, and this child needs an operation, an *appendectomy* to remove her appendix.

Appendicitis is a common occurrence in children. The appendix is a narrow, fingerlike projection that hangs off the *cecum*, the end of the large intestine. It is a sort of blind pouch, a hollow tube that opens only into the large intestine. It has no function that we know of, although there are some clues as to what it was once for. The main clue is that large animals that eat plants, such as horses, have a huge appendix. It appears to be an important organ of digestion for them. Perhaps as humans evolved to a more mixed diet, the appendix was no longer needed. At any rate, we no longer need it; now it can only cause us trouble, although the majority of people still go through life without any problems with it at all.

Appendicitis begins when the narrow opening of the appendix gets plugged up. A common cause of this is a hard fleck of stool that, by bad luck, gets wedged into the orifice of the appendix. Another potential cause is swelling of the tissues around the appendix that squeeze it shut, swelling such as from a nearby infection. What happens next is that the bacteria inside the appendix—there are billions of them because it is connected to the large intestine—start to grow and multiply inside the now sealed-off appendix. The appendix, as well as the tissues around it, becomes inflamed. That is the point at which the child's abdominal pain becomes localized to where the appendix is: the right lower quadrant of the abdomen. If the process continues, such as if a diagnosis is not made and a surgeon does not take out the appendix, the appendix bursts open and dumps infected material into the abdomen. When that happens—a ruptured appendix—the child may need more extensive surgery to fix things. But the situation is still quite fixable.

It is not always easy to diagnose appendicitis in its early stages, especially in very young children, who cannot tell you about their symptoms. The main clues here were the fever, the progression of the pain from vague, generalized pain to sharp localized pain, and the loss of appetite. If the doctors are unsure of what is going on with a child with potential appendicitis, sometimes the child needs to be admitted to the hospital for close observation to see how things go. Often an imaging study, such as a CT scan, is needed to sort things out.

CHECKLIST AND ACTION PLANS FOR DIGESTIVE AND ABDOMINAL PROBLEMS

Abdominal complaints are very common in children. Unlike with URIs, the possibilities range from the trivial to the very serious, so parents play a key role in sorting out what to do. This checklist will help you focus your thinking. As with the lists in the previous chapters, if you are unsure of what to do, it is reasonable to move your action plan up to the next category. This chapter does not have a "Call 911" option because the chances of abdominal complaints being that much of an emergency are extremely low. On the other hand, if your child is severely ill and you have no way of getting him to the emergency department, that is always an option.

Watchful Waiting

1. Your child is drinking fluids well.
2. If vomiting is present, it looks like what your child ate.
3. Your child is making roughly normal amounts of urine.
4. Your child's abdominal pain is mild.

Call the Doctor

1. Your child is not drinking as well as you would like.
2. Your child does not seem to be making the usual amounts of urine.
3. Fever is present along with the abdominal complaints.
4. Your child is vomiting bile (greenish-yellowish material).
5. Your child's abdominal pain is moderate.

Take Your Child to the Emergency Department

1. There are signs of significant dehydration: your child's mouth and tongue are dry; she makes few tears when she cries; her output of urine is reduced; the soft spot on her head appears more sunken; she is extremely listless.
2. Your child is vomiting blood or there is blood in the stool.
3. Your child's abdominal pain is severe no matter its location, especially if accompanied by fever.
4. The abdominal pain is sharp and localized to the lower-right part of the abdomen, especially if there is also fever and loss of appetite.

5. Vomiting is so severe that your child can keep nothing in her stomach (this needs to be somewhat age-adjusted: older children can tolerate this situation far better than younger children or infants).

7

BUMPS AND CONKS ON THE HEAD

Rare is the child who gets through childhood without hitting his head many times on things. There are several reasons for this. First among them is that children are adventuresome. Toddlers are absolutely fearless in the way they wander aggressively into any place or situation that captures their attention, and their confidence far exceeds their coordination. Older children ride bicycles, climb trees, and jump down from garage roofs. Even though these things are a normal part of childhood, they also can lead to injuries— scrapes, bruises, cuts, broken arms, and the occasional conk on the head. This chapter is about the last one: head injuries.

Toddlers are especially prone to hitting their heads on things. This is not only because of their bumbling incoordination. It is also common because, relative to their body size, a toddler's head is larger than that of an older child or an adult, so the chances of banging it on something when they trip and fall is higher.

Even though most head bonks are trivial, leaving only a passing lump on the scalp, a few are quite serious. In fact, among children who suffer serious, life-threatening, or even fatal accidents, head injury is a prominent underlying cause. So parents of children who hit their head have good reason to be concerned. As in our previous chapters, the best way to begin your understanding of how doctors evaluate head injuries is know a few things about how the brain works both in normal conditions and following any sort of injury. Along the way, it is also good to know something about the spinal cord and its attached nerves since children can hurt those too.

The brain is arguably the most important organ in the body, so the body protects it carefully with an excellent armor casing: the skull. Adults have solid skulls surrounding their brains. The only openings are a series of small holes for various nerves to exit the brain, such as those to the facial muscles and the eyes, and one very large hole at the base of the skull for the spinal cord to pass through and continue its course down through the spinal column of the back bones.

Infants and toddlers have somewhat different skulls than older individuals. Their skull bones are thinner and are also still growing. Since their brains are still growing too, the surrounding skull needs to expand to allow for that growth to happen. A baby's skull is made up of several plates of bone separated from each other. This allows the skull to make more room as the brain gets bigger. These plates touch each other along boundaries called *sutures*, which you can feel with your fingers. You also can feel the spot at the top of the head where several suture lines come together. The technical name for that is the *anterior fontanel*, but non-physicians call it the *soft spot*. The soft spot of an infant is often quite large. If you push on it you are fairly close to touching the brain itself, which lies beneath a couple of layers of thin tissue.

After brain growth is complete, the sutures fuse together, completing the protective armor casing of the skull. This happens surprisingly early in life; the brain of a first-grader is about 90 percent as large as it will be when she is an adult. Head growth after that is mostly from other parts of the head, such as the facial bones and the sinuses. Sometimes one or more of the sutures fuse too early, a condition called *craniosynostosis*. This may require surgery to re-open the gaps between the bone plates, but surgery isn't always necessary because the brain is able to adapt quite well to the new situation. Even if it can adjust, though, the surgery may be done for cosmetic reasons because otherwise the child's head will not grow symmetrically.

The front part of the head contains the sinuses, those air-filled cavities above and below the eyes and behind the nose. You read about those back in chapter 4. Infants have almost no sinus cavities yet because these structures enlarge with age. As you also read in chapter 4, sometimes the sinuses can be a source of problems if they become infected, but overall they are useful to have because without them our skulls would be much, much heavier to carry around on our neck. Even though the front of the skull has a great deal of air in it from the sinuses, the bones that surround the brain are quite solid.

The skull is not the only protection the brain has. Inside, nature has devised additional protection. The brain does not simply sit inside the skull; rather, it floats. If you could look inside the skull, you would not immediately see the brain. Instead, you would see a tough, white membrane called the *dura*. The dura completely surrounds the brain (and the spinal cord too). The dura is essentially a fluid-filled bag, floating inside of which is the brain. The fluid compartment between the layers is called the *subdural space*. This space is filled with clear *cerebrospinal fluid*, or CSF for short. This provides important protection because the fluid that fills the dura acts as a shock absorber when the head is struck, absorbing some of the energy of the blow.

The brain is also covered by several layers of membranes, together called the *meninges*. The inner membranes are tight against the brain. They are very delicate structures, in contrast to the outer layer, the dura, which is a tough, fibrous sheath. The meninges encase the brain and spinal cord, extending all the way down the inside of the spinal column to its base above the hips. Outside the dura is the skull, and outside that are several layers of muscles before we reach the skin and hair.

As you will read, there are limits to the ability of the shock-absorbing system of the skull and CSF to reduce injury. The system of skull and CSF works very well for protecting the brain from low-velocity, glancing blows. It does less well for direct impact, high-velocity ones. The brain can also be injured when the brain gets shaken inside its fluid compartment. This is a common form of injury. The blow sets up a shock wave that jostles the brain in the CSF, driving it against the side of the skull opposite the blow. The result can be injury to the other side of the brain when it strikes the hard, inflexible skull.

The spinal cord is connected to the base of the brain and exits the skull through the large hole at its base. It is surrounded by the same dura and also floats in CSF. It is protected by the bones of the spinal column, although, unlike the skull, this is not a solid wall of bone. The spinal cord ends at about the level of the middle of the back, but the dural sac extends all the way down to the tailbone. This is extremely useful to physicians because we can sample some of the CSF at the level below where the spinal cord stops, a procedure known as a lumbar puncture or spinal tap. Since CSF circulates throughout the dural compartment, testing the CSF at the base of the back gives us important information about what is happening around the brain, especially if we suspect infection. You read a little about spinal taps in chapter 3; you will learn even more about this common pediatric procedure in chapter 12.

Another aspect of skull and brain anatomy that is very important for understanding the effects of conks on the head is the blood circulation around the brain. This is because one of the more-serious things we worry about with head injury is bleeding inside the skull. It is uncommon, but the consequences can be severe.

Inside the dural sac, the brain is closely covered with a delicate series of membranes. There is a meshwork of veins that course their way through the fluid-filled gap between the dura and these inner layers. A blow to the head can cause these veins to be injured, and if that happens they bleed into the dural space. A common mechanism for this is a shaking of the brain inside the skull. What can happen is an acceleration then a deceleration event as the brain is bounced around. This can shear one or more of the delicate veins.

There is another network of blood vessels outside the dura, traveling between the skull and the dura. The largest of these are arteries, not veins. Since arteries carry blood at a much higher pressure than veins, the blood inside them comes out faster if they are broken. So if one of those arteries is injured, the resultant bleeding is brisker than it is for the subdural veins.

Bleeding from one of the subdural veins is called a *subdural hematoma*, and that from one of the arteries just outside the dura is called an *epidural hematoma*. Many of these injuries do not require anything besides careful watching in the hospital (we do not send children with them home from the emergency department), but some cause life-threatening emergencies requiring emergency surgery to fix. Why is that?

A good way to think of the skull is as a rigid, closed box. An infant with open sutures does not have such a rigid container, but their skull is still constricting enough to make the analogy valid for them too. If the pressure goes up inside the box, then the brain gets pushed on, or squeezed, and that can damage the brain if the pressure persists or gets worse from swelling of the brain or continued bleeding from injured blood vessels. The only way to relieve the pressure is to do an operation to relieve the pressure. Sometimes, if the pressure is rising quickly, that operation needs to be done in an emergency fashion. Delay can be catastrophic.

So this is the dilemma for parents, and for doctors too. Conks on the head are common. Most of the time, in fact the overwhelming majority of times, the injury is trivial because the brain has good protective mechanisms. Once in a while, though, the injury is serious. How can a parent decide if a fall from a bicycle or tree bough requires a trip to the emergency department or even a call to 911? The case scenarios in this chapter will show you how a doctor thinks about these injuries. With the brain, the stakes are high, so we always should err on the side of caution. But any parent can gain a working, practical knowledge of how we sort these injuries into those that are innocent, those that are concerning, and those that are dangerous.

Before we do that, however, we need to talk about the ways that doctors look at the brain, how doctors image the contents of the skull. This is because the bottom-line question for many children whose parents bring them to the emergency department following a head injury, and who are not obviously injured seriously, is whether or not the child needs tests to look for serious things.

The most common way to image the skull and brain is using radiation, or x-rays. The traditional study was a simple x-ray of the skull. This will show broken bones, that is, skull fractures, but it will not really tell us anything about the brain itself. For this reason, simple skull x-rays are not used that much any more. A better kind of x-ray is a CT scan. It shows the brain itself. It is very good at showing if there has been any bleeding inside the skull or if there is anything pushing on the brain to increase the pressure. It also shows the skull bones better than simple skull x-rays, which is another reason we no longer use the latter test very often.

If CT scans are so useful at seeing inside the brain, why not do them on every child who comes to the emergency department with a head bonk? After all, this is the brain we are talking about and the stakes are high. The answer is that the amount of radiation exposure from a CT scan is significant, much higher than that from simple x-rays of the bones or chest. Researchers have become increasingly aware of the possible risks of that radiation, especially for children. One recent research study estimated that, in years to come, approximately one in four thousand cancers will be the result of diagnostic radiation, the majority of it coming from CT scans. The reason this is particularly important for children is that radiation risk is cumulative over a lifetime, so children, with so much of their life ahead of them, are at higher risk.

My goal here is not to scare you about the risks of CT scans. Properly used, they are life-saving. The best way to think about it is to know that everything we do in medicine carries risk—everything. If we choose to do nothing, that decision carries some risk too. We are always weighing what we call the *risk-benefit ratio*, the risk of doing something balanced against the risk of not doing something. Yes, CT scans carry some risk, although it is tiny. We must consider, though, the risk of not doing a CT scan. If the benefits of doing the scan outweigh the risks from doing it, then we should do it. But this also means we should do our best to avoid the scan if possible. Every doctor seeing a child with a head injury is weighing the pros and cons in this manner.

There is another way to image the brain, one that carries no risk of radiation. It is called a *magnetic resonance imaging scan*, or MRI for short. This technique is esoteric compared to x-rays and it is difficult to explain briefly how it works, but it uses a powerful magnet to detect how the various molecules in the body respond to changes induced in their behavior by the magnet. The result is a series of amazingly precise images. Bleeding and pressure on the brain are easily seen, as well as many other things.

If MRI has no radiation and gives such detailed pictures, why should we not use it on all children with head injuries? Why do the CT? One practical reason is that MRI scanners are not as abundant as CT scanners—it is a complicated and expensive technology. For children especially there is another problem: MRI scanning is very slow. A simple CT scan of a child's head can be done in a matter of seconds. In contrast, an MRI scan takes twenty minutes or so at least. This difference has practical consequences for children because for both scans you must hold very still or the image is blurry.

Most children, even an active toddler, can hold still for the few seconds of a CT scan. I have yet to meet the toddler who can hold perfectly still for a twenty-minute MRI, and many school-age children find that nearly impossible too. Even adults are often intimidated by the close confines and very loud noise of the MRI machine.

This means children getting an MRI scan must usually be given sedative drugs to make them hold still. Often they need to be completely anesthetized. This deep sedation carries risk, such as a slowing down of breathing. We have standard ways of dealing with that possibility, but my point is that the need for deep sedation, and for recovery from the sedation drugs, often offsets the advantage MRI has through its lack of radiation. Once again we are back to the risk-benefit ratio: we balance the risk of doing the test against the risk of not doing it, of not getting the information it yields.

Now that these important preliminaries are out of the way, we can get down to what we can learn from specific scenarios.

WATCHFUL WAITING

One evening your ten-year-old is running too fast down a long flight of wooden stairs to the basement. He trips, and tumbles head-over-heels down to the bottom, striking his head on the floor. You hear the crash and find him sitting on the floor. He is a little dazed, but he can tell you exactly what happened, although he scoffs at the suggestion he was running too fast. That is, he has full memory of everything immediately before and during his fall. Afterward he complains of a headache for an hour or so, and he has a lump on the back of his head that is a little tender to the touch. You are concerned, but you think he is probably fine. A few minutes later he is completely alert. Should you take him to the emergency department at this point? Does he need any x-rays or scans of his skull and brain?

One of the most important things we use to assess what to do with a child with a head injury is what the child does immediately after the injury, then some minutes after that. We also pay attention to what we call the *mechanism of injury*, the circumstances of what happened. An example of a concerning mechanism of injury is a fall from higher than six feet or so; the higher it is, the higher our concern. An example of a still more concerning mechanism is a high-impact injury, such as from an automobile accident.

But even though we consider the mechanism of injury, the most important thing is still what the child does and how he looks afterward. What we are looking for is any alteration in mental status. By that we mean confusion, disorientation, or memory loss. The memory loss can be quite brief, only a minute or so. That is why memory of the entire event is a good screening tool; if the child recalls everything, including landing on his head, then his memory is fine.

This is a good time to talk about *concussions* because whether or not this child may have had one is important. Everybody has heard the word, but when doctors use it we mean something quite specific: a concussion is defined as a brief loss of normal brain function. The most common function affected is short-term memory. The usefulness of short-term memory in injury screening is related to the way the brain processes and stores memory. It uses more than one area to do this.

Short-term memory, your recollection of what has happened in the previous fifteen minutes or so, is stored in one place; long-term memory is stored somewhere else. Your short-term memory is continually collecting information on the front end of your consciousness, while on the back end your brain is moving out your experiences of the past few minutes to a more secure storage area. The system for short-term memory is a bit fragile, and memories are not secure until they are moved to a more stable site. This is why people with subtle memory problems often exhibit their difficulties through their inability to keep track of what just happened to them, even though they can recall more-distant events just fine.

A good analogy for this process is the random-access memory, or RAM, of your computer. The RAM can be wiped out by a power surge or a power outage on your computer. Unless you have saved the information to your hard drive or other device, the information is lost. Think of short-term memory in your brain as similar to RAM in that way, with the brain's more stable storage site being like your hard drive. A concussion often wipes out a few minutes of your brain's RAM. It is common after a concussion for the person not to recall the injury, and often to have lost a bit of memory of what came before it as well. Asking a child what is the last thing they remember before the injury is a good way to screen for that.

There are other symptoms often seen with a concussion besides memory loss. Vomiting and persistent headache are common. Visual disturbances, such as blurry or double vision, can happen. In the hours or even days following a concussion, a child may have these symptoms or others, such as difficulty concentrating, continuing headaches, or labile emotions. Of course none of these later symptoms help a doctor or parent decide in the moment if the child has experienced a concussion.

By definition a concussion shows no abnormalities on a CT or even MRI scan. But the symptoms clearly indicate the brain has been injured in some way, even though our scans are not sensitive enough to pick it up. Isolated concussions heal, and the child is fine afterward. Our main concern is the effect of repeated concussions. Of particular concern is if a child experiences another concussion before the symptoms of the first one have passed. Recent research, especially with professional athletes like football players, has shown there is a significant chance of long-term consequences to the brain from repeated concussions that follow close on each other.

What do we do for a child with a concussion? The answer is simple: we observe them closely to see if they are getting worse. That means doing some very low-tech things, such as asking them where they are, asking them to count, and doing simple checks of their vision. Further deterioration after a concussion, such as brain swelling, is very uncommon, but if it is happening we can always be alerted by changes in the child's mental status, his state of alertness. The parents of a child who has experienced a concussion are given explicit instructions about what to watch for and told to return promptly if they see anything changing.

Now let us return to this child who fell down some stairs. Afterward he was completely alert and aware and had full memory of what had happened. He has a mild and passing headache from hitting his head and he has some swelling on his scalp, as you would expect. Because he has normal mental status and no concussion symptoms, you can safely watch this child at home, and he certainly does not need any scans of his brain.

If you are a bit unsure of what to do, there would be nothing wrong with bumping this case up into the "Call the Doctor" category. As with all the actions plans and checklists in this book, if you are sitting on the fence, it is best to move up into the next category.

CALL THE DOCTOR

For this scenario, imagine that the boy from the last scenario, complaining about the pain from the bump on his head, sits down to dinner. An hour later, he complains of some nausea and then vomits. He is still alert in every way, but he feels nauseated. He still has a headache, only now he says that more than just the region of the bump hurts; now his pain is more generalized. It is evening and in a couple of hours it will be his bedtime. If this were your son, it would cross your mind that he might have some other reason for nausea and vomiting, the flu perhaps, but he seemed fine earlier in the day. You would not be surprised that the bump on his head hurts, but now his headache seems more than that. If you were in this situation, what should you do? Might he have a concussion in spite of his good memory of the event?

This scenario is intended to show you that the boundaries of the categories we doctors use for evaluating head injuries are often fuzzy. They can overlap, and sorting things out can require experience and judgment. This child's situation lies in the grey area between confidently observing him at home and clearly needing a doctor's evaluation. No book like this one can give the guidance you would need to sort things out safely. So if this child were your son, it would be best to call the doctor for some advice.

GO TO THE EMERGENCY DEPARTMENT

This scenario features an eighteen-month-old child. She is playing on a screen porch about six feet above the ground. She manages to push out the screen at the bottom of the door, and she then falls down six concrete steps, striking her head on the way down. She has some scrapes, but no significant breaks in the skin. She cries immediately after it happens. Her mother finds her just afterward. The child seems groggy and disoriented, unsteady on her feet. Then she vomits. What should the mother do? Should the child be taken to the emergency department? If so, is it safe for her mother to do so herself, or should she call an ambulance?

This case is an opportunity to put into practice some of the principles we were talking about in the previous case. But before we even get to an assessment of this child's symptoms, note that the mechanism of injury of this accident, a fall from six feet above the ground, is a sign we should not shrug this off but recognize it as having a good possibility for significant problems.

The next thing to note is that this is a young child. In our discussion about concussions we laid considerable emphasis on using confusion, disorientation, and brief memory loss as clues to what might be serious and what is probably not. This child is not preverbal, but she certainly is not old enough to describe things for you. Because of that, if this were your daughter, you should have a lower threshold for taking her in for an evaluation. The doctor will not be able to communicate with her any better than you can— probably worse, because you are the parent—but he can do a detailed examination. He also has a CT scanner, of course.

Looking at this story, it is likely the child suffered a concussion. She was groggy and she staggered around immediately afterward. This tells us she was confused, disoriented, uncoordinated, or all of these things. She also vomited shortly after she fell, something that is also common with concussions. The combination of all these things—mechanism of injury, confusion and grogginess, vomiting—suggests concussion. This case is best evaluated in the emergency department by an expert, not a parent. Your daughter may need a CT scan. She even may need to be admitted to the hospital overnight for observation.

Watching a patient closely over the succeeding hours after a head injury like this is far and away the most important part of that patient's care. Often this can be done by parents, but it is best to do it after a doctor's evaluation and under the guidance of a physician. The younger the child, the more difficult it is for a parent to do this on their own. But that is something for you and the doctor to discuss.

The final question for this case is how to get to the emergency department. Since this child is now reasonably alert and interactive, it would be appropriate for her parent to drive her to the emergency department herself.

CALL 911

For this scenario, imagine the same child is in her parents' bedroom on the second floor and she manages to push out the window screen, after which she falls through the window and lands on her head. Fortunately she hits earth and not concrete. As with the scenario above, other than a scrape there is no break in the skin on her head. The child moves around on the ground just after the impact, really more like thrashes about, and does not really wake up and cry for several minutes. What should her mother do in a situation like this?

The clear answer, one that most any parent would probably give, would be to call 911 for help. There are several good reasons for this, but the main one is that paramedics will bring expertise and equipment with them essential to transporting the child safely. While waiting for the ambulance to come, what should this child's parent do? The child is lying quietly. She is breathing fine. She moves around a little when her mother stimulates her by calling out her name or pinches her. Should her mother, for example, scoop her up and carry her inside the house? If you find yourself in a situation like this, the best answer is to leave her where she is, if you can. If it is not possible, then move her as little as possible. Why is that?

The main reason to minimize disturbing her is the possibility that she may have injured her neck. Compared with adults, or even older children, neck injuries that affect the spinal cord are very uncommon in toddlers. This is probably because the bones and neck tissues in toddlers are in some way more resilient, such that the same mechanism of injury affects small children differently. But such injuries can happen, and a fall from some height and landing on the head is a concerning mechanism of injury for the possibility of spinal cord injury.

The spinal cord runs down through a series of holes in the vertebral bones, the bones of the neck and back. These bones give it some protection from injury, but they can be broken or displaced from their normal position, potentially injuring the spinal cord. For a fall from some height that lands a child on his head, the most vulnerable is the cervical spine, the neck. The bones themselves can be broken. It is also possible for the soft tissues around the spinal column to be stretched such that they no longer support the neck bones as they should. The result of either of these rare events is what we term an *unstable spine*. You want to move the neck as little as possible until it can be supported artificially. The paramedics have simple support devices, such as a collar they can put around the outside of the neck and a firm carrying board, to make sure the spine remains stable until the possibility of injury is evaluated by the doctors in the emergency department.

What is happening inside this child's brain is that she has experienced a significant concussion, one that has made her at least briefly unconscious. In spite of all the Hollywood movies you might have seen where one character neatly knocks out another, it is actually quite unpredictable what kind of blow to the head will cause this. For example, I have cared for children who fell from third-story windows, landed on their heads, and then got up and walked away. I have cared for others who got concussions from falling down a few carpeted stairs. This is why, although mechanism of injury is important, looking at the child afterward is the most important thing.

As you read above, a concussion will heal. The major concern for this child is that she has injured her brain from the fall, such as bruised its surface when the brain floating in the cerebrospinal fluid banged against the inside of the skull. She may also have experienced one of the kinds of bleeding events you read about. There are also other, more-serious possibilities. The bottom line is that this child needs to be taken promptly to the emergency department by skilled paramedics who know how to do the transport safely.

CHECKLIST AND ACTION PLANS FOR BUMPS AND CONKS ON THE HEAD

Mild head injuries are common in childhood, and nearly all the time they are of no consequence. But sometimes they are serious. Most of the serious ones are obvious from the beginning, and it is clear that the child needs medical attention. But of great concern to parents, and to physicians too, is that sometimes an injury may seem innocuous at the beginning but then evolve into one that is not. That is the worry. This chapter is intended to help you find your way through that dilemma. The brain is a fragile organ, and you should certainly err on the side of caution.

Watchful Waiting

1. The mechanism of injury is trivial, such as a fall of less than three feet.
2. Your child has complete memory of the injury.
3. Your child has no other symptoms, such as nausea or vomiting.

Call the Doctor

1. The mechanism of injury is more significant, such as a fall from three to six feet.
2. You are suspicious, but are unsure if your child is having concussion symptoms or not; or your child has a single mild symptom such as headache.

Go to the Emergency Department

1. The mechanism of injury carries a higher potential for problems, such as a fall from over six feet.

2. Your child has memory loss.
3. Your child is too young to question, or he shows signs suggestive of confusion or disorientation.
4. Your child has symptoms of persistent vomiting or headache.

Call 911

1. Your child has a sustained decreased level of consciousness after the injury.
2. Your child experiences a convulsion after the injury.
3. Your child has abnormal neurological signs after the injury, such as an inability to walk or move an arm or a leg.

8

SPRAINS, DISLOCATIONS, AND BROKEN BONES

Children bump and bang themselves a lot. In the last chapter you learned about one of the more potentially severe examples of this: blows to the head. But of course children also bang other parts of their body, especially arms and legs. These injuries can be as minor as bruises, but they also can include more severe things like broken bones. Less severe are the sprained wrists, ankles, and knees that are especially common in sports. Any emergency department waiting room has its share of children waiting to see the doctor for these sorts of problems. Do all of them need to be there, especially in the late evening or nighttime? This chapter will help you decide if that trip to the emergency department is necessary right after the injury, a bit later, or ever.

There are about 206 bones in the human body. The exact number varies a little because some people lack a trivial bone or two and others have an extra one. These bones are of several kinds. Some are flat, like the ribs and the skull. Others are long bones, such as in the arms and the legs. Still others are short, even round, such as the bones in the wrist, ankle, and spine. All of the bones, especially in children, are hollow. This is a good thing because otherwise the weight of the skeleton would be quite a burden to haul around. This is why birds have very hollow bones; they need to be as light as possible.

Bones may seem simple, just hard chunks of inert material, but this is not the case. The skeleton is as alive as anywhere else in the body. It is in fact a busy place, with many jobs to do. The most obvious job is to support the body in space, serving as the scaffold that holds us up. But bones have other important tasks as well.

The inside of a bone, the *marrow*, contains the cellular factories where blood cells are made. As we age the proportion of the marrow that is actively involved in making blood cells becomes less, but in children most of the bones do this to some extent. Surrounding the marrow is the hard part of the bone, called the *cortex*. What makes it hard is a calcium salt called *hydroxyapatite*, a substance that makes up at least half of the bone's material. Surrounding the cortex, on the outside of the bone, is a layer of tissue called the *periosteum*. It has an important role in nourishing the bone.

If you think about it for a minute, a child's skeleton has a problem to solve. It must be a hard framework for the child's body, but it must also grow with the child. That inert, hard scaffold must be constantly modifying itself to get bigger. Nature has an ingenious way of solving this problem.

At the edges of the bones of children there are regions known as *growth plates*. For a long bone, such as in the arm or leg, there are growth plates at either end of the bone. In these areas cells are actively making new bone so that the bone can grow longer. These are important structures since damage to them can affect, even prevent, further growth of the bone in that spot. Broken bones, or *fractures*, that involve the growth plate can therefore be tricky to handle. Once a child reaches adult size, these growth plates go away.

Of course as a child grows that child's bones must not only grow longer, they also must get fatter and wider. The body does this using a process of active remodeling. Like a homeowner who is never quite satisfied with the house, bones, even in those areas in the middle of the bone away from the growth plates, are constantly demolishing older bone scaffolding and erecting new. To make the bone grow wider, special cells on the inside, lining the marrow, are continually absorbing away the hard cortex. Meanwhile, a different set of cellular workers is laying down new bone on the outside. The result is that the bone can get wider and the marrow cavity can grow larger. This same cellular growth-and-repair crew is what heals a broken bone.

What happens when a bone breaks, how do we know it has happened, and what do we do about it? The simplest fracture to describe is a break through one of the long bones, such as an arm or leg bone. When that happens, the cortex is typically, although not always, snapped through on both sides of the bone, leaving two free ends. The periosteum, the membrane covering the bone, is generally intact. A *closed fracture* (or *simple fracture*) means that the bone ends stay underneath the skin; an *open fracture* (or *compound fracture*) means one or both of the bone ends break through the skin. Any parent knows an open fracture needs the immediate attention of a doctor, so for our purposes we are more interested in closed fractures. These need a doctor's attention too, but the issue for parents is when to suspect that a closed fracture has happened.

Children have more limber bones compared with adults, so fractures of their bones also come in other varieties besides bones completely broken through. One of these is often called a *green stick fracture*. The analogy is to a small branch fresh off a tree. If you bend it, the branch often will only suffer a break on the surface opposite the side you are bending and will not break completely through. Children's bones can do this too. Children also may have what is called a *buckle fracture*, which is really a variant of the green stick fracture. In this type of fracture, the bone is not broken through, but the site is disrupted, buckled, in a characteristic way.

In these situations, the key point is that there are not disconnected ends of the bone at the fracture site.

What makes us suspect a fracture? The mechanism of injury gives a clue, since a trivial bump, for example, is unlikely to break anything. After that, the most suspicious thing is any deformity, such as crookedness of an arm or leg. These cases are usually obvious and not likely to cause parents much trouble in deciding what to do. A more subtle fracture sign is localized tenderness. This means a specific spot over the bone that hurts significantly when you push on it with a finger. It is more than a diffuse soreness; it is pain over a discrete spot. After an hour or so a fracture site generally begins to swell. Thus a doctor would suspect a fracture if there was an injury that made it possible, plus tenderness and swelling at the spot.

How do we diagnose a fracture? The answer is the only way to see the bones is with an x-ray. An x-ray shows the ends of the broken bones. It also generally shows less-severe injuries, such as buckle fractures, in which there are no broken ends. The x-rays need to be taken from more than one angle because a single picture only shows two dimensions; it is possible to have a fracture but not see it if only one x-ray view is done. The multiple views are also important because if there are broken ends, the doctor needs to define the relationship of the ends to each other, and that takes more than two dimensions.

Once a doctor identifies a fracture, how does he fix it? The first key principle is that to heal, the broken ends of the bone need to be brought close to one another and oriented in approximately their normal position. The alignment does not need to be perfect because the body is good at fine-tuning the alignment as the bone heals. The second principle is that the fracture ends need to be held immobile against each other for several weeks to heal. If the ends are allowed to move around, they will be continually damaging the new bone forming, and the fracture will not heal.

What we do specifically depends upon the fracture. A broken arm generally needs a cast to hold the ends immobile and near each other. Even a buckle fracture should have some sort of cast or splint to protect the area while it is healing. A broken skull bone, however, does not need anything because the fractured surfaces are naturally held in place by the tissues of the head and scalp. The exception to this is if one edge of the skull bone is pushed down, depressed well below the other edge. Similarly, a fracture of a pelvic bone generally stays in good alignment and usually only requires that the child rest until it heals.

Some of the pain from a fracture comes from the inflammation in the area, but much of it comes from movement of the free ends of the broken bone. Once the ends are immobilized with a cast (or sometimes other means), the child's pain gets much better. Buckle fractures, by definition, do not have any loose ends. But they do hurt. This pain is lessened by protecting the area with a splint or cast, so we usually do that. Fracture pain is significant, and many children will need potent painkillers, such as an oral narcotic like hydrocodone or oxycodone, for a day or so.

The bones need to be connected together to work as a unit. This is the job of the joints, which are regions where one bone meets another. The body has several kinds of joints that allow movement in defined directions. Hinge joints like the knee or the fingers allow back-and-forth motion in one direction only. Other joints, like the ball-and-socket joints of the shoulder and hip, allow more variety in movement. There are also joints that allow only minimal or hardly any movement at all. Rib joints are examples of this category. There is some wiggle possible where the ribs meet the breastbone in the front and the spine in the back to allow for movement of the ribcage when we breathe, but the extent of this is small. The joints of the pelvis bones allow very little movement, since that part of the body requires a strong, rigid frame to support us.

Since bones are hard, it would not work for the ends of the bones to grind back and forth on each other as they moved. To make things smooth, joints include a bag of fluid that lubricates the area of the bone ends and allows nearly frictionless movement. Some joints, such as the knee, also have soft tissue pads that cushion the spot where one bone meets another.

The joint fluid bag requires something sturdy to hold it in place between the bones. The joint *ligaments* perform that function, and they also stabilize the joint. Ligaments are tough bands of fibrous tissue that surround joints and support the bone scaffold. They tie joints in place by connecting to the bones on either side of the joint. Although they are made of tough, gristly tissue, they also can stretch to some extent. They need to do this to allow normal joint movement. But they can be overstretched and in that way injured, which is what a *sprain* is, or they can be torn when a too-strong force is applied to them.

Sprains are common. How do we diagnose and treat them? In particular, how can we be sure there is no fracture present? There are some very common sprains for which we have criteria to help us decide. Ankle sprains, for example, are particularly common. The most common mechanism is a child leaping in the air and coming down on a foot that is twisted inward. For these injuries the doctor can often rule out a fracture after examining the ankle. For some sprains, though, the only way to tell that a swollen, bruised joint area does not contain a fracture is by doing an x-ray.

We treat sprains with a plan that carries the acronym RICE. This stands for rest, ice, compression (such as with an elastic bandage or tape), and elevation. The components of this therapy move healing along using simple principles. Resting the injured area prevents reinjuring it; cold reduces swelling by dampening the effects of inflammation, especially immediately following the injury; mild compression and elevation reduce swelling by reducing fluid accu-mulation in the tissue. It is difficult to slow down an active child, so in general they can be allowed to do whatever activities they like if they feel comfortable doing it. Acetaminophen or ibuprofen helps with the pain. Ibuprofen also reduces inflammation.

Sometimes children can suffer what is called a *joint dislocation*, although with the exception you will soon read about, these are relatively uncommon. A dislocation happens when the alignment of the bone ends in the joint is disrupted such that the ends no longer sit in the correct spot and the joint cannot function normally. Nothing is broken, but the bones need to be relocated, or put back into alignment.

There is a particular dislocation injury seen in preschool children that is good for parents to know about because it is common. It happens in the elbow, and it is sometimes referred to as *nurse-maid ' s elbow* or *babysitter ' s elbow*. It is a dislocation at the end of the radius, one of the bones in the forearm, on the end nearest the elbow. There is a ligament that ties together the two arm bones just below the elbow. This ligament can be injured and the end of the radius pulled out of position. The most common cause is pulling hard on a child's straightened arm, so it is not a good idea to swing your toddler by his hands with his feet off the ground or to yank vigorously on his outstretched hand. It is painful to a child when it happens, but it is nearly always easy to fix by manipulating the arm in a specific way to guide the end of the bone back into place. Any emergency department physician experienced in caring for children knows how to do this.

How do we detect and treat joint dislocations and sprains? The answer is that the signs and symptoms are very similar to those of a fracture, only occurring over a joint. There is localized tenderness and swelling. Often an x-ray is needed to make sure no bone is broken, but this depends upon the circumstances. A dislocated joint may appear obviously out of alignment. If there is no fracture, we generally manage sprains with the components of the RICE program. Dislocated joints need to be manipulated back into place.

Support of the joint with a brace of some sort often helps, particularly with the knee. Severe sprains and joint dislocations can take several weeks or more to heal—as long as a fracture takes.

A child can also injure a muscle severely enough to make a parent wonder if the injury requires a trip to the emergency department. These injuries are usually to the larger muscles in the body, particularly those in the leg. Muscles are tied to the bones with either ligaments or tether cords called *tendons*. An easy tendon to feel is the *Achilles tendon*, the one in your heel, which connects your heel bone to a muscle in the back of your calf. The tendons on the back of your hand are also easy to feel; they connect the muscles in your forearm to your hand bones.

The way we move a particular body part is to contract a muscle, which pulls on the tendon connecting that muscle to an adjacent bone. Thus we flex our knee by contracting the muscles in the back of our thigh and straighten it by contracting muscles in the front of the thigh. Muscles often come in paired teams such as that, with one opposing the other.

Muscles can be injured by a direct blow to them or by being stretched beyond their usual limit. When that happens, some of the muscle fibers are pulled apart and may even tear. The signs of a pulled or torn muscle are tenderness to the touch and swelling, only in this case the tenderness is not over a bone or a joint. There also may be some discoloration of the area from a bruise inside the muscle. The treatment is generally the same RICE program, plus time and over-the-counter painkillers as needed.

Before we get to this chapter's specific scenarios, there is an important principle to discuss about injuries of this sort: a great many of them are not emergencies. Of course if a child falls from a piece of playground equipment and immediately has an arm that hurts, swells, and looks crooked, that is likely a fracture and the sooner the fracture ends are put in alignment and immobilized, the sooner the child will feel better. But doing that will not by itself make the arm heal any faster. If your child has an injury that you may think could be a sprain, a pulled muscle, or even a fracture, and if the symptoms are not severe and there is no deformity, much of the time it is appropriate to observe what happens over the hours following the injury to see if it gets better on its own.

Now that you know these general principles, we can get to the specific scenarios.

WATCHFUL WAITING

Your twelve-year-old son falls off a tree limb six feet above the ground. He lands on his outstretched right hand. He comes into the house saying his wrist hurts. You have a look at it. It is not swollen and he can move it around just fine. He is right-handed, and he is able to use that hand reasonably well, although he says it hurts. You check on him an hour later and he is using the hand to play a video game. It still aches, he says. At this point should you take him to the emergency department for a wrist x-ray?

A fall from some height onto an outstretched hand is an extremely common mechanism for breaking a wrist. What is typically broken are not any of the wrist bones themselves, which consist of eight small, roundish bones packed into the region between the end of the forearm and the first series of hand bones. What gets broken is one or both of the forearm bones just before their joints with the true wrist bones. So the chances of this child breaking a bone are significant.

In this case, though, other than the mechanism of injury there is not much to suggest any broken bones. There is no swelling of the area and nothing looks out of alignment. There is no *point tenderness*, meaning that although the child's wrist is generally sore, there is no spot that really hurts when you push on it with your finger. There are a few other things any parent could do to check it out. You could find that he can wiggle his fingers just fine and this does not make the pain worse. You could ask him to squeeze your hand, finding that he can do that with normal strength and without much change in the pain.

Another important thing in this scenario is that a few hours later his pain is much better and he is using his hand normally. So there is nothing here, other than the mechanism of injury, that suggests a fracture. You can safely watch this at home. If any of the things noted above appear, you can safely have the wrist checked out later. Meanwhile you could give him an over-the-counter painkiller, such as acetaminophen or ibuprofen. If the wrist had been broken, however, this is a good time to talk about how it would be fixed, because if a child came to the emergency department with a fracture like that, it would be fixed right then using a technique called *closed reduction*.

The first thing the doctor, most likely an *orthopedic surgeon* (a bone surgeon), would do would be to give the child something for the pain. This is generally a drug like morphine, a narcotic painkiller, given in a vein through an IV. Depending upon the situation, more powerful sedatives are often used in addition because a closed reduction hurts quite a bit. Moving the ends of the bones around against each other is painful.

The doctor then generally injects a painkiller—similar to what a dentist uses when drilling teeth—that acts locally to numb the area around the fracture. He then takes a firm hold of the bones on either side of the break and brings them back into line. Typically this involves pulling the ends apart, tipping the hand, and then flipping the edges together. The alignment does not have to be perfect because the bone ends have the ability to fine-tune their orientation to each other as they heal. An x-ray then verifies that everything is right.

To keep the newly aligned ends in place, the doctor then applies a cast. Plaster went out years ago; now we use fiberglass that comes in rolls and hardens quickly after it is made wet. It is much lighter and more durable than plaster. (It also comes in a wide variety of colors, which children enjoy.) The trick with putting on a cast is to make it neither too tight, because that would pinch the arm and possibly cut off circulation, nor too loose, which would allow the bone edges to move and prevent good healing. Sometimes the area is too swollen to put the final cast on at the time so the area needs a redo a couple of days later when the swelling has gone down.

WATCHFUL WAITING

Now imagine the same son of yours is playing basketball. He leaps for a rebound and, rather than landing squarely on his feet, comes down on the outside edge of his foot, with his ankle turned inward. He has immediate pain and limps off the court. An hour later he is still limping, but he can bear weight on his leg. Yet another hour later he is still limping around, so you take his sock off and have a look. Compared to his other ankle, the injured one is a bit swollen. There is a little purplish discoloration. Could this be a broken ankle, or is it just a sprain?

This scenario is overwhelmingly likely to be a sprained ankle. The key observation here is that although your son is limping, he is able to bear weight on the ankle. That is virtually never the case if a bone is broken. But even if there is a crack in one of the ankle bones, there would be no harm in waiting through the night to see how things go. If his pain and swelling are no better or even worse in the morning, you can have him seen then. Meanwhile you could use a RICE program and give him acetaminophen or ibuprofen for the pain.

A child with a severely sprained ankle, one that prevents him from walking, is worth having evaluated in the emergency department, perhaps the next day. After ruling out a fracture, either by examining the ankle or by an x-ray, the doctor can fit him with an ankle brace and crutches to help him get around while the ankle heals.

CALL THE DOCTOR

There is not much a doctor can tell you over the telephone in situations like those we are considering in this chapter because an actual examination of the injured area is the most important thing. However, if you are looking at your child and you are unsure of what you are seeing, it may help to get some advice from an experienced person to guide you. This may be particularly helpful with a young child, such as a toddler, who cannot tell you anything.

GO TO THE EMERGENCY DEPARTMENT

You are shopping with your two-year-old daughter. She is at that age when riding in the stroller all the time is no longer fun. She wants to walk around. She darts around a rack of merchandise and you grab her right hand to pull her toward you. She cries out and immediately seems to be holding her right arm funny—she holds it straight and stiff against her body, thumb side in. She also refuses to use the arm. What should you do? Should you watch her overnight and see if it gets better? After all, you did not pull that hard. How could anything be broken?

This child has nursemaid's elbow, the condition you read about earlier in the chapter. It is a form of dislocation of the end of the radius, the thumb-side bone in your forearm. But even if she did not have that particular problem, there are several clues that would tell you that watchful waiting is probably not the best way to handle this one. The main thing is that this child refuses to use her arm at all, holds it in an unusual way, and experiences worse pain when you move it.

This particular injury is generally quite simple for an experienced doctor to fix quickly. No painkillers are needed; distraction techniques are usually sufficient. The doctor takes hold of the child's hand and then smoothly rotates the palm of the hand upward while he flexes the elbow using his other hand. The end of the radius nearly always pops back to its proper place. Generally no x-ray is needed. In fact, it is a well-known phenomenon that if you send a child like this to the x-ray department, she often will return moving her arm normally. This is because while positioning the arm for the standard two x-ray views, the technician frequently carries out the maneuver I described above and unknowingly fixes the problem.

CALL 911

This vignette is a tale of two baseball players, both running to catch a foul ball. They collide at high speed and both fall to the ground. One player gets up rubbing his shoulder but can move his arm around fine. The other one cannot get up, or even move much, because the upper part of his left leg is excruciatingly painful and rapidly swelling. What should be done with him?

It is the milder injuries that can puzzle parents about what to do. This one is easy, and any parent would be pretty sure that the second child has broken his leg. In fact, he has broken his *femur*, the largest bone in the body, which goes from the hip to the knee. When this bone gets broken, it can cause other problems besides a simple fracture.

For one thing, the marrow cavity of the femur is large, and when the bone is fractured a large amount of blood can escape into the surrounding tissues. For another, the femur is surrounded by some of the most powerful muscles in the body, the muscles of the upper leg. When the femur breaks, these strong muscles typically go into spasm. That often pulls the broken ends of the bones so that they overlap by an inch or more, making closed reduction impossible. And even if it could be done, there is no easy way to put on a cast to hold the bone ends in place. That is why this kind of fracture requires surgery to fix. Often the orthopedic surgeon will place the leg in traction first. This means attaching a device to the ankle that steadily and gradually pulls the whole leg downward, relaxing the muscles and bringing the bone edges closer to alignment.

There are several surgical techniques to fix this kind of fracture with what is termed an *open reduction with internal fixation*. The technique the surgeon uses depends upon the circumstances and exactly where in the bone the fracture is. A common technique is to run a thin metal rod down the marrow cavity, joining the ends together and keeping them aligned while the bone heals. Other times the fracture requires a metal plate screwed into the bone edges to keep them together.

This is not a situation in which a parent should attempt to bring the child to the emergency department in their car. The leg will be extremely painful to move in any way, so you cannot carry this child anywhere. Paramedics will have a cart on which to lift him and then roll him to the ambulance. They are experienced at stabilizing the leg while they do this. Also very important, the paramedics carry powerful painkilling medications they can give to the child through an IV.

CHECKLIST AND ACTION PLANS FOR SPRAINS, DISLOCATIONS, AND BROKEN BONES

If an injury causes severe or persistent pain or obvious deformity, then the child needs to be evaluated by a physician. Most parents understand this. The difficult question is what to do with milder, less dramatic injuries. What general principles can parents use? One key principle is that moderate or mild injuries can nearly always be observed to see how the child does; you are not putting your child at risk by waiting to see how the symptoms evolve.

Watchful Waiting

1. The pain is not severe and steadily improves after the time of injury.
2. Your child is able to put some weight on the injured area.
3. Your child is able to use the injured area to some extent.
4. There is no deformity of the injured area.

Call the Doctor

1. Moderate pain persists without improvement after twelve hours.
2. Swelling and local tenderness appear no better after twelve hours.

Go to the Emergency Department

1. Your child is unable to bear any weight on the injured area.
2. The pain is more severe, it is not improving, or it is worsening.
3. Swelling of the injured area is persistent or worsening.
4. There is obvious deformity of the injured area.

Call 911

1. Your child is unable to move after the injury.
2. Movement after the injury causes severe pain.

9

CUTS, LACERATIONS, AND OTHER SKIN INJURIES

The skin is the thin envelope that surrounds and protects the organs of the body. It has several crucial functions, one of which is to keep body moisture in. This is important because one of the largest components of our bodies is water. When this ability to keep water inside is compromised, such as from a large burn, water loss can be huge. The skin also keeps harmful elements of the surrounding environment out. It can stretch significantly when needed, which is a good thing. If it could not, we would find it impossible to move our arms, legs, and fingers very far. We also could not laugh or smile easily.

But the skin is much more than a passive barrier, more than a flexible armor that keeps our insides in place. In fact, the skin is best thought of as a separate organ of the body, one just as active and important as the metabolic factory of the liver or the reliable pump of the heart. It makes things too—important things for the ongoing health of the body. For example, the skin is a key participant in the immune system. It contains specialized cells that can recognize enemy invaders, such as germs, and mobilize the body's defenses to fight them. It has other cells that make *melanin*, the pigment that helps protect us from the sun's ultraviolet rays. The skin is a busy, busy place.

Resilient as it is, the skin is also easily and commonly injured. It is tough in some ways, but extremely vulnerable in others, which is a price we pay for its flexibility. Insects and lobsters have tough outer shells to protect their insides, but they can only bend in a few places. Humans and other mammals have a much more complicated covering.

Another reason skin commonly gets injured is easy to see—there is a lot of it. It has a huge surface area. This is particularly so for children, for whom the ratio of their surface area to their internal volume is large compared with adults. The skin is the outer boundary of the body, our frontier with the outside world. So unless it comes through the mouth or nose or anus or genitalia, any agent that seeks to injure the body first encounters the skin.

For these reasons emergency department doctors care for many children with skin injuries. Cuts and scrapes, for example, break through the barrier. But the skin can be injured in other ways besides encountering a sharp object. A blow from a blunt object can result in a bruise. Or the skin can be injured by heat and cold. There are still more ways than these in which the skin can be hurt, such as rashes and inflammations, things you will read about in the next chapter. This chapter is about traumatic skin injuries. To understand how we care for those, you need to learn something about the structure of the skin. It may look like a simple envelope, but as you will see, it is actually a complicated and fascinating organ of the body.

The skin is built in layers. The outermost layer, which carries the fancy name of *stratum corneum*, is not really alive. It is made up of dried-up cells that form a tight moisture barrier. These cells begin their lives deeper in the skin, although still not very far down. As the dried-up cells on the outermost surface get shed off—something that happens constantly—younger cells work their way up from below, ultimately taking their place on the boundary to the outside world. For an individual cell, this journey takes around two weeks. You can see the process happening if you examine the back of your hand with a magnifying glass. This region of the skin is called the *epidermis*, a term simply meaning "on top of the dermis."

The *dermis*, sometimes called the *dermal layer*, is next. It is a complex community of several kinds of cells. Many of these cells manufacture the physical components of the skin, substances which give the skin its flexible and elastic nature. Think of the skin cells as embedded in a meshwork of microscopic fibers, a scaffold with struts and girders running in all directions. A key component is *collagen*, something you have probably heard of if only because it appears in cosmetic commercials on television. Collagen is the soft, springy stuff you feel when you pinch yourself. There are also elastic fibers there, which help give skin its ability to stretch in any direction and then spring back afterward.

Our skin is hairy, although more so in some parts than in others. The hair shafts are embedded in the dermal layer. At the base of each hair is a *follicle* containing cells that replace the substance of the hair as the hair grows up and out in a manner similar to the cells migrating upward in the epidermis. Also like the outermost skin layer, a hair is made up of material that is not living cells.

Besides being hairy, our skin is also sweaty and greasy, although once again these properties vary from place to place on our body surface. The cells that make these important, although sometimes annoying, substances also live in the dermal layer. They are organized into *glands*, tiny factories manufacturing these fluids, with small tubes running from each to carry its product to the skin surface.

Both sweat and the greasy stuff, called *sebum*, are important for our health. Sweat is a key component in our heat-control mechanism. Evaporation of sweat from the skin draws heat away from the body. One way we know this is that rare individuals who cannot sweat, or who are taking medications that interfere with sweating, can dangerously overheat. And without natural oils to lubricate our skin, it can become cracked and dried out, interfering with its important barrier function. This happens to some extent anyway, especially in areas exposed to harsh conditions, which is why skin lotion feels so good on rough, chapped skin.

The skin is rich in other kinds of important cells. For example, it has a dense network of nerve cells, particularly those that convey pain and touch. Imagine for a moment what would happen if we did not have these. It certainly hurts when you prick your finger with a pin. But if you did not have such pain sensors, consider the effect of touching a red-hot stove. Instead of the minor burn that would occur during the split second between your initial touch and then pulling away your finger, you would have a severe burn from prolonged contact. People who have deficient pain sensation are continually at risk for severe injuries.

The fine-touch nerve sensors of the skin are also crucial to our ability to do what we do every day. These nerves are found everywhere in the skin, but certain areas are extraordinarily rich with them. Our fingertips are one such area. This allows us to do all those delicate things with our fingers that we take for granted every day.

Since the skin is injured frequently, it needs a good repair mechanism. So living throughout the skin are cells whose job it is to clean up injured or damaged tissue. A cut in the skin needs to be mended, its edges joined together again. There are skin cells standing by to do this when necessary. The result does not always restore the skin exactly to the way it was; a scar is the handiwork of the repair cells. A scarred area does not have the complicated architecture of normal skin, but it reestablishes a continuous, protective shield.

As you can see, the way to think about the skin is not as a simple barrier. Instead, think of it as a bustling place. Because it is so busy on the cellular level, it needs a good blood supply. The blood brings needed oxygen and nutrients to the skin cells, allowing them to go about their tasks. The skin therefore has a dense network of blood vessels, a fact made obvious when you scratch or cut yourself. This is what gives your skin its pink color, if you are a white person. If you are darker pigmented, you can still see the effect of this lush blood supply by looking at the palms of your hands.

What happens when the skin gets injured? A scratch is an easy example to consider. A trivial scratch involving only the epidermis, the outermost layer, leaves a mark but does not bleed because it did not penetrate to the tiny blood vessels, the *capillaries*, lying in the dermis. This sort of minor injury may leave only a red mark on the skin. The redness is from increased blood flow to the area since, even though the injury has not broken through to the dermal blood vessels, it still injures the tissues a bit, which causes inflammation, and inflammation draws an increased blood flow to the area. A deeper scratch or cut, if it reaches down to the dermis, may bleed a little bit because it breaks some dermal vessels, but that bleeding stops quickly.

A deeper cut, what we call a *laceration*, goes right through the dermis and reaches the tissues beneath it. These so-called *subcutaneous tissues*, meaning "tissues beneath the skin," contain blood vessels larger than capillaries, and if one of those is cut there is more bleeding than comes from just the capillaries of the skin. There also is a significant amount of fat in the subcutaneous region, though more in some areas than others. If you look at such a laceration, you can often see yellowish globs of fatty tissue peeking out. A laceration can be even deeper, and of course more serious as a result. What tissues get affected depends upon where the laceration is. There might be muscles, tendons, nerves, larger blood vessels, joints, or even bones involved.

Before we get into specific examples, it is useful to know some of the general principles doctors use in treating scratches, cuts, and deeper lacerations. Children heal very well from the vast majority of these injuries, but the injuries should be managed correctly from the beginning to make this happen.

A scratch or cut that does not penetrate all the way through the skin does not need a doctor's attention, as most parents know. What it needs is to be washed clean and protected while it heals. This is because the cut breaks through the skin's protective barrier, and the outside of that barrier is normally covered with bacteria. The great majority of these cause no trouble to us, even if the skin surface is broken. There are several varieties of bacteria, though, that are notorious for causing infection if given the chance. Chief among these is one that carries the fancy scientific name of *Staphylococcus aureus*, or *staph* for short.

Staph can take advantage of tiny breaks in the skin, disruptions so small we can barely see them. Sometimes staph can even invade through normal skin openings. For example, it can find its way down a hair shaft or sweat gland to cause infections like boils. So if there is a visible break in the skin barrier, and the population of staph on the skin is sufficiently high, a local infection can result. This can easily be prevented, however, by using some simple measures. The most important of these is just washing the area with soap and water. That dramatically reduces the size of the bacteria population. The germs will return, but meanwhile the tissues of the area of the cut get a head start at healing and reestablishing the skin barrier. After the cut is washed, a thin film of antibiotic ointment, available over-the-counter, can help to keep the bacteria at bay for a bit longer, but that is typically not really necessary.

A simple adhesive bandage can protect the cut while it heals, especially during the few hours it takes nature to make her own bandage for the area—a scab. Since the skin has such a good blood supply, a cut makes it bleed. You can help the bleeding stop by applying pressure with a cloth, but most small cuts stop bleeding on their own because the skin has its own way of managing the situation. Any tiny vessels that get broken are quickly plugged through a process in which blood particles called *platelets* have an important role. The body's blood-clotting mechanism cooperates with the platelets to make the other principal component of a scab, which is a meshwork of microscopic fibers. Once the scab is formed, the tissues beneath it heal, shedding the scab when the healing is done. If you pick off a scab before that process is finished, the cut will bleed again.

Cuts that go all the way through the skin to the subcutaneous tissues below, true lacerations, will also generally heal if we do nothing besides keep the area clean, especially if they are small, but the final result would not be satisfactory without some assistance from us. When the skin is cut through, the repair cells on one side of the cut cannot cooperate with the repair cells on the other side over the gap because the distance is too far. If we did nothing to help that, the tissue would heal by filling in the gap with scar tissue rather than with normal skin. The result would be a substantial scar, accompanied by a depression in the surface if the laceration is of any significant size, say a half-inch or so long. The laceration would also be more likely to become infected with bacteria since there is a larger break in the protective skin barrier. So these kinds of injuries need a doctor's attention to heal the best. What do doctors do to manage them?

Treating a deeper laceration begins the same way as treating a minor cut or scratch: we clean the area thoroughly. We wash the skin area around the cut with germ-killing soap. We also clean down in the laceration itself to get out any infected material. To do this we do not just daub it with a wet cloth; we irrigate it thoroughly with *saline*, a solution having the same concentration of salt as the blood. Because the saline is germ-free, or sterile, it carries away most of the bacteria; those few left behind can be taken care of by the skin's natural defense mechanisms.

To do the job well requires a lot of saline. An average-size laceration may take a pint or more, depending upon the circumstances. A cut with a relatively clean, sharp object is handled differently than a cut obviously contaminated with dirt. Cuts sustained in particularly dirty environments, such as a farmyard, call for a large amount of irrigation solution. What we do is fill a syringe with saline, gently wash the saline over and down into the wound, and then repeat. Before we quit washing we take a good look inside the wound to make sure there are not any bits of grit or other foreign material. Once the laceration is clean, it is ready to be closed.

When we close a laceration, we want it to heal leaving as small a scar as possible. The first step to accomplishing that is the cleaning part, because any infection will inhibit healing and worsen the scarring. The next step is to bring the edges of the cut together until they gently touch. What we want is to approximate proper alignment of the edges without causing any tension in the tissue.

If the laceration just goes through the skin and does not gape open too far, we have several choices. The standard technique is to suture, or stitch, the skin edges together. It is a method that is thousands of years old. Ancient doctors used a needle and linen thread. These days we use synthetic thread made from nylon or something that resembles monofilament fishing line. These threads, already joined to a curved needle, come in sizes from stout to barely visible. The finest thread is used for the face, the more sturdy for other areas, such as the leg. After numbing the skin with an anesthetic, the doctor passes the needle entirely through the skin into the subcutaneous area on one side of the cut, brings it out through the skin on the other side, draws the two edges together, and secures the stitch with a knot. Additional stiches are needed at quarter- to half-inch intervals, depending upon the site.

Straight lacerations are simple to close. In contrast, crooked or jagged ones can be challenging. For all of them, though, the principles are the same: bring the wound edges together as best you can to where they were before the injury and seal the edges snugly, but not too tightly.

If the laceration is a deep one, going well into the subcutaneous tissues, the wound often needs to be closed in layers, starting with the deepest part. This is important for reducing the tension at the surface level. For one thing, deeper wounds tend to gape open more, and to pull together the edges of the skin with just a surface suture requires more force. So instead we use stiches down in the deeper tissues to bring them together first. This takes the tension off the subsequent surface stiches, allowing the skin edges to come together easily.

Surface stiches need to be taken out after the cut has healed. How long they need to stay in varies with location. Face wounds usually can have their stitches out in five days or so because the area heals very quickly. For other areas of the body, the stitches need to be left in place for seven to fourteen days. They should not be left in any longer than that because the stitch holes themselves will leave a scar of their own. The stiches used below the surface, those times when the wound needs to be closed in layers, do not need to come out. They are made of material that dissolves away and is absorbed by the body.

Once the skin edges touch, the repair cells that live there can join them together permanently. When that happens, the result is always a scar, a line of tough connective tissue that is not normal skin. As you have read, there are several things we do to minimize the size of the scar, but there will still be one. Most emergency department doctors are very good at laceration repair, but extensive or unusual lacerations may require the specialized skills of a plastic surgeon. Whether or not that is needed is a judgment call involving several considerations, one of which is if such an individual is available.

We have other ways of closing lacerations besides sewing them. Some wounds can be sealed using a device with metal staples. The apparatus looks very similar to a tool you might buy in a hardware store. This is often done for lacerations in the scalp. Other lacerations, particularly ones in which the edges naturally fall together, can often be joined with glue. The glue, which is also similar to material you might buy in a hardware store, lasts as long as it takes for the edges to heal. This technique can be helpful for small cuts on the face in young children. Finally, we also have strips of special tape that sometimes can be used to approximate the edges of a wound. However, the problem with these is that they can slip, allowing the wound edges to separate a bit. If that happens, the gap will result in a larger scar.

Now that you know something about the general principles of how we handle skin injuries, it is time to consider our case scenarios in detail. We do not have a "Call the Doctor" category in this chapter since a laceration is a difficult thing to describe over the phone. Of course you can do this if you are unsure and want some general advice, but that advice is hard to give without the doctor seeing the injury. On the other hand, technology may be allowing this to happen soon. I have cared for several young patients with skin injuries (and rashes) of which their parents had taken a picture with a cell phone and sent it to me to look at. Perhaps we will see more and more of that in the future.

WATCHFUL WAITING

Your four-year-old is running around with a ballpoint pen in her mouth. She trips, falls, and bangs the inside of her mouth with the pen tip. She cries, and you see blood running out of her mouth. You help her up and rinse her mouth with water to dilute the blood. You then have a look inside with a flashlight. You see a flap of tissue hanging off the inside of her cheek, slowly oozing blood from underneath it. The gouge underneath the tissue flap is perhaps a quarter-inch deep at most. Does she need to go the emergency department for this?

Our discussion earlier in this chapter was all about the skin, its component parts, how it is injured, and how it heals. But children also frequently get injuries inside their mouths. It is not uncommon for a parent to be confronted by a scenario like this one. The key point here is that injuries inside the mouth are different. The surfaces of the inside of the cheeks and gums are not really skin. We call them *mucosa* because they do not have the same layers as the skin.

Mucosa injuries like this one heal quickly by themselves. In fact, the tissues inside the mouth are some of the fastest healing of any tissues in the body. They have a lavish blood supply, which is a key reason they heal so fast and why they virtually never become infected in spite of all the bacteria that normally live in the mouth. It is also the reason they can bleed quite a bit. But if the bleeding stops, as with this child, a gouge out of the cheek the size of the one this child has does not require any medical attention.

Very large or deep cuts inside the mouth sometimes need to be closed with stitches, especially if the bleeding continues, but the majority of them do not need this. Lacerations that start on the inside of the mouth but then extend out to include the skin of the lip should be seen by a doctor because this is an area where a scar can be quite noticeable—you want to make the scar as small as possible.

For the child in this scenario, you could put an ice cube in her mouth to keep the swelling down and help with the pain. If you are unsure of what to do, of course, it is best to go to the emergency department.

GO TO THE EMERGENCY DEPARTMENT

Your one-year-old has just learned to walk. Like all children at that stage, she falls down a lot, especially when she tries to run. This evening she is hurrying around your living room coffee table and stumbles, hitting her head on the corner of the table just above her eye. She is naturally upset afterward, but she is alert. You first hold a clean cloth against the area for five minutes or so to slow the bleeding. Then you have a look at the injury. It is about a half-inch long or so, lies just above her eyebrow, and is oozing blood. You can see skin edges gaping open a bit. What should you do?

This particular injury—a small laceration around the eye or on the forehead from colliding with the corner of a piece of furniture—is quite common in children. I have cared for many children just like this one. The edges of the wound are separated enough for you to see that it goes down through the skin. Although this one would heal on its own, it is best to close it to avoid a noticeable scar on the face. So you should take her to the emergency department.

The tissues of that part of the body generally come together quite easily and heal very fast. Depending upon the exact orientation of the cut, the doctor may suggest using tissue glue to close it. If his suggestion is to use stitches, it will probably take about three stitches, and he will use very fine suture material, typically of the kind that looks like fishing line. Facial stitches do not need to be in place as long as those on other body parts, as noted, so these will need to come out in about five days. This is an important point since, as I also noted above, leaving stitches in too long will cause a small scar just from the stich holes. This is a particular concern on the face.

Sewing skin hurts, so before the doctor can use sutures he will need to numb the area with a local anesthetic. That makes this a good time to talk about the options we have for doing that. For many lacerations, the standard medicine to numb the skin is lidocaine, which is similar to what a dentist uses to numb the gums before working on teeth. It does have to be injected with a needle, and it does sting as it goes into the tissue. We can reduce a child's discomfort by using a very small needle and by injecting slowly, but it still hurts for a few seconds until the area is completely numb.

For small lacerations on the face we have another option besides injecting lidocaine. Because the skin of the face is so thin it can directly absorb many medications easily. For cuts like this we often can wet a cotton ball with one of several anesthetic mixtures and hold it against the cut for several minutes, after which the area is sufficiently numb for the child not to feel the needle of the stich going in.

Children, especially preschool children, are frightened by the whole experience of getting a laceration repaired. So another aspect of caring for any child needing a laceration closed, but especially a toddler like this one, is to consider what options we have for giving the child sedative or anti-anxiety medications before we start. This not only makes the experience less traumatic for the child, it also results in a better repair because when the child is comfortable the doctor can concentrate on getting every stitch in just the right spot.

GO TO THE EMERGENCY DEPARTMENT

Here is another example. Your eleven-year-old son is doing some woodworking and the utility knife he is using slips and slices open a two-inch gash on the inside of his forearm. He presses a cloth on it and comes to show it to you. Before looking closely, both of you take the prudent step of sitting down first. For those not used to looking at these injuries, the first glimpse can make you queasy indeed. You cautiously peel back the bloody cloth and see a laceration that gapes apart at its middle. The wound goes right through the skin and you can see yellowish globs of fatty tissue showing.

You quickly replace the cloth and appropriately head for the emergency department. What can you and your son expect there?

This scenario is of a straightforward deep laceration. The laceration needs to be inspected carefully, washed out, and closed. This is a good spot to pause and answer the question of timing. With a laceration like this, assuming the bleeding has stopped, how much time does a parent have to get it taken care of? The standard limit on the time a laceration can go without repair is twenty-four hours, although most would say under twelve hours is much better. As a general rule, if a wound is older than twenty-four hours it is best not to sew it completely shut because the odds are high that the wound will become infected. This is because the bacteria in the area have had a long head start. Like everything in medicine, there are exceptions—a very clean wound, for example, might be safely closed. It is a judgment call by the doctor.

If an older, contaminated laceration cannot be closed, how is it treated? The answer is that it is thoroughly washed out, inspected for bits of debris (which are removed by washing or with an instrument that looks like a tweezers), and then often packed with sterile gauze, depending upon how deep the laceration is. A dry dressing then covers the area. This dressing is regularly changed, and the wound will usually need to be seen by a doctor several times as it heals. And it will heal, but from the inside out, a process termed *healing by secondary intention.* Because the skin edges are never joined together, the healing will leave a large scar.

What care can the child and his parents in this scenario expect when they get to the emergency department? The first thing will be a gentle inspection and washing of the area. Since the wound hurts, we usually postpone the thorough, deep washing until we have numbed the area. For this sort of injury, that means injecting lidocaine up and down the wound edges. Once the area is completely numb, the doctor can wash it out with saline and have a good look at the inside of it.

We already know there are bits of fat visible through the wound, indicating that the laceration penetrated to the subcutaneous tissue. What the doctor needs to determine is if the knife injured any important structures down there, such as nerves, muscles, tendons, or blood vessels. Since the bleeding has stopped, injury to a large blood vessel is unlikely, but there are other important things in the forearm. As you get closer to the wrist, these are quite near the surface. So the doctor needs to shine a bright light down in there and see. He will also test for potential injuries to these deeper structures by having the child squeeze his hand and by testing sensation in the hand and fingers. If all those are fine, the wound can be closed. If there are potential problems, then a specialist, such as an orthopedic surgeon, needs to check things out first.

Once the wound has been inspected and cleaned, it is time to close it. This one will need to be repaired in layers because it is well through into the subcutaneous tissue. The deeper layer will be repaired with an absorbable suture material. The skin-surface stitches will be made with material that needs to be removed in seven to ten days.

Suture removal is done with a small forceps and scissors. The doctor (or nurse) first grasps the end of the stich material and gives it a tug to lift the knot above the skin. The stich is then snipped with the scissors beside the knot, after which a quick pull with the forceps removes the stitch. The process does not hurt, although the child will feel a bit of tugging.

CALL 911

You are cooking dinner in the kitchen and your three-year-old is playing on the floor. He is an active child and you watch him carefully out of the corner of your eye. But in spite of your diligence, his curiosity and lightning-quick moves manage to pull a saucepan of hot soup off the stove and onto his lower face and chest. The area is bright red immediately, and you soon see several blisters on his neck. You also notice that his lips are rapidly swelling since some of the soup caught him there. You realize that he has a significant burn, one that needs medical attention. How should you handle this scary situation?

This scenario is our opportunity to talk about burns. These injuries are common in children, particularly scalds from hot liquids. Many parents remember from first-aid classes that we commonly classify burns in increasing order of severity as first-, second-, or third-degree burns. Physicians now generally speak of *superficial*, *partial thickness*, and *full thickness* burns, although you will still hear the earlier terms frequently. The newer classification makes sense because it describes the skin injury: just the top (superficial), into the dermal layer (partial thickness), or entirely through the skin (full thickness).

How we manage burns depends on the severity of the burn and its location. Burns such as the one in this scenario are typically of mixed type. For example, they may be superficial in some places and partial thickness in others. This child already shows evidence of that, with some areas being only red (superficial) but others having blisters (partial thickness). Another important point is that, particularly for more severe burns, it may be difficult to classify the burn accurately right away—it can take a day or so to tell.

This child has some partial-thickness (second degree) areas, but most of his burn is superficial (first degree). Why should his parent call 911 and not bring the child to the emergency department herself? The reason is that this child has burns around the mouth, and his mother has already noticed some swelling of his lips and tongue. That swelling will undoubtedly get worse before it gets better. The concern in this scenario is that the swelling might get in the way of his breathing, even block his airway. For that reason, it is best to get the paramedics there quickly because they have the tools and expertise to deal with that problem if it happens.

Another example of a scenario in which you should call 911 is a burn associated with a flash, such as from lighting a barbecue, in which your child may have inhaled heated air. Accidents like this can burn the inside of the child's airway and cause serious swelling of the tissues that could interfere with breathing.

Once such a child reaches the emergency department, his burns will be treated in several ways. The burn areas themselves, particularly the partial-thickness areas with the blisters, will be cleaned and then dressed with an antibiotic cream. As you learned earlier in the chapter, the skin is an important moisture barrier. When the skin is burned to any significant extent, a child needs additional fluids, typically through an IV. Burns also hurt much more than any other skin injury. So another important aspect of this child's care will be to give him painkillers, also usually intravenously at least at first, to control his pain. Most likely this child will be admitted to the hospital at least for a day or so until his fluid and pain needs are taken care of and the possibility of airway swelling is gone.

CHECKLIST AND ACTION PLANS FOR SKIN INJURIES

For skin injuries, a parent's options are somewhat more limited in that the choice of "Call the Doctor" is less likely to be helpful simply because it is difficult to assess these injuries over the telephone. As with previous chapters, if you are unsure of what to do, advance to the next level.

Watchful Waiting

1. A cut does not go deep enough into the skin to make the edges fall apart.
2. The bleeding is easy to stop with only direct pressure.

3. A burn or scald is red with no blisters, is small in size, and does not involve the face around the mouth or nose.
4. A sunburn has no blisters, and your child is drinking well.

Call the Doctor

1. You are not sure of what you are seeing in a cut.
2. You are unsure if a red burn is too extensive to manage at home.

Go to the Emergency Department

1. A cut is through the skin with the edges gaping apart.
2. You see other tissues, such as yellowish fat, at the bottom of the cut.
3. A scald or other burn is more extensive or involves the face around the mouth or nose.
4. A burn is blistered.

Call 911

1. You cannot control the bleeding of the cut with pressure alone.
2. A burn is extensive (if unsure, it is best to call 911 for help).
3. A burn involves the face around the nose or mouth or was caused by heated air or gas.

10

RASHES

The last chapter was about mechanical injuries to the skin from sharp or hot objects. The skin can be injured in other ways. Rashes fall into that category too, if you think about it. They represent the skin's response to a wide variety of noxious things, ranging from infections to poison ivy, insect bites, or a particular brand of soap.

Children get a lot of rashes. There are several reasons for this. One is that children, compared with adults, have very sensitive skin that can be easily irritated by things in the environment. Another reason is that children get relatively more viral infections than adults do, and viral infections are a common cause of rashes.

Very few rashes require a trip to the emergency department; many do not even need a trip to the doctor's office. However, there are a few important exceptions to this general rule. Mixed in among all the rashes children get are a few that are signs of serious illness, and these should be evaluated promptly by a doctor. Fortunately there are fairly easy ways to identify these more-serious situations. This chapter will tell you how physicians evaluate rashes and what makes us suspicious that a serious problem may be present. The chapter will also tell you about many of the common rashes of childhood—helpful information for any parent to have.

One of the interesting things to know about rashes is that evaluation of them is one of the last areas of medicine to resist the invasion of diagnostic tests and scans; we mostly diagnosis rashes the old-fashioned way—by looking at them and often feeling them with our fingers. Certain rashes do lead us to do some tests because we know those particular rashes are often associated with other problems. But those things are generally secondary to making the diagnosis. The key thing is just looking at the rash and interviewing the parent to get some information about how and when the rash started.

Doctors divide rashes according to a set of categories. Some of these are based upon what the rash looks like, others relate to what the cause is. These distinctions have fancy names that it is not worth your while to read about. But some of the attributes that define the categories are useful for a parent to know because understanding them will help you decide what to do with your child if she has a rash. They are also helpful categories because it will allow you to describe the rash over the telephone or tell a doctor more precisely how your child's rash may have evolved over time.

The first category concerns color. Most rashes are reddish-colored to some degree. That is because inside the individual rash spot there is usually a component of inflammation, and inflammation makes red blood cells gather in the tissue from the skin's tiny blood vessels. So the area is pink to red-colored. Of course the color of the rash depends to some extent upon the underlying color of the skin. So if your child has a dark complexion, the red color will be less obvious. A few rashes are purple-colored rather than red. They look like tiny bruises because, in effect, that is what they are—areas of the skin where the smallest blood vessels have broken and are oozing blood into the skin.

Some rashes are flat on the skin; if you close your eyes and run your fingers over them you cannot tell they are present because there is nothing to feel. Other rashes consist of small bumps you can feel above the skin surface. Sometimes the bumps are solid, and at other times they may have little fluid-filled caps on top of each bump. The fluid, if present, can be clear or cloudy. These caps can break open and weep the fluid out onto the skin. When the fluid dries, it leaves a crust, which is why these kinds of rashes often have scaly, crusted areas.

There is also size to consider. Some rashes consist of tiny spots, others have larger blotches or a mixture of sizes. Often the rash spots stay in one location, but sometimes a rash can seemingly magically move from place to place on the body over a short span of time. A series of tiny spots may coalesce into larger spots or blotches.

Finally, rashes vary in what symptoms they cause the child. From a practical standpoint, the main distinction for us is between rashes that itch and rashes that do not itch. A few hurt when you push on the involved area, but not many.

When a doctor looks at a rash, she is running this descriptive catalog through her mind because what the rash looks like, accompanied by a conversation with the parent, is the main criteria she will use to decide what the cause is. A parent can easily learn a few of these principles and put them to good use.

The majority of rashes in children are small red spots that do not move anywhere, do not have any fluid on the top of each bump, do not hurt, and do not itch. The chest and abdomen are common locations. These kinds of rashes are often caused by viral infections. If your child has a rash like this, a clue would be the presence of other symptoms of a virus, like fever, vomiting, or diarrhea. Sometimes, though, a rash like this just comes out of the blue without any other symptoms. What should you do about it? The answer is little or nothing. You certainly do not need to trek into the emergency department unless your child is ill in some other way that would bring you to the hospital even without the rash. If the rash is sufficiently itchy to bother your child, you can apply an over-the-counter anti-itch cream, such as hydrocortisone. But most of the time no therapy is needed.

We also commonly see this sort of rash if a child is having a reaction to a medication. Any medicine can cause a rash, but amoxicillin and its cousin Augmentin are notorious for doing it. Both these medicines are commonly prescribed for ear infections. Since ear infections are common as well, being the most frequently diagnosed condition in children, doctors encounter this rash frequently. Several other oral antibiotics also cause rashes. So if you see a rash suddenly spring up on your child, recall any medicines he has recently taken. If your child gets a rash like this and is taking a prescribed medication, particularly an antibiotic, call your doctor to see if he wants to make any changes in your child's medications. We do not always change the medicine, however, since in some cases the rash fades away even if the child continues to take the medicine.

Another common childhood rash is *hives*. This kind of rash is quite different from the first one, even though hives can be caused by a reaction to a medicine. Hives are nearly always a reaction to something in the environment. Once in a while this is a germ of some sort, but usually it's something the child ate, breathed in, or touched.

Hives are larger in size that the first rash I described, ranging anywhere from a half-inch or so to over an inch in size. They usually are pinkish in color, rather than red, and they swell upward from the skin and make a bump. They often move around; new ones appear and old ones fade as quickly as over the course of an hour. Most importantly, hives usually itch. The prototype for what a hive looks like is an insect sting. Although most hives do not hurt like a bee sting, that is what they look like.

Hives are caused by a different mechanism than the first rash you read about—the small, red spots. Hives are caused by the release into the skin of a substance called *histamine*. The skin is full of special cells that contain this material and are primed to release it when triggered by something. Histamine makes the blood vessels of the skin leak fluid, which is where the swelling comes from. Histamine triggers the itching too. Often you can just ignore the hives and wait for them to pass, but sometimes they are important to treat, even in the middle of the night.

The most important consideration is if the hives are accompanied by any problems in breathing, such as wheezing. You can judge such problems using the same criteria you learned in chapter 5 about breathing troubles. Of most concern is the rare situation in which the hives occur inside the mouth, causing swelling in the back of the throat or tongue. This situation needs prompt attention in the emergency department. If there are any breathing problems at all, a 911 call is indicated.

We treat hives with one or more of several medications that improve the itching symptoms and make the hives shrink. Diphenhydramine (Benadryl, many others) is available over the counter and is quite safe. It comes in both liquid and capsule form, and the appropriate dose for your child is on the container. If the hives are severe enough to affect breathing or cause airway swelling, we use several injectable medicines in the emergency department. Ambulance paramedics also carry these medications if your child is having breathing problems.

Another common, itchy rash is *contact dermatitis*. This rash is red, sometimes raw-appearing, and may have small blisters. Contact dermatitis is caused by something irritating the skin, such as poison ivy exposure. *Diaper dermatitis* in infants and toddlers is caused by irritation of the skin around the groin area; this one may be complicated by having the raw skin secondarily infected by germs, typically yeast.

There are some skin infections that look like rashes. The most common one is called *impetigo*. It is usually caused by the same germ that causes strep throat. This bacteria can sometimes be found on the skin, and when present it can invade through the outer layer of the skin if that layer gets disrupted in some way, such as by scratching. Strep germs can also make their way into apparently normal skin. The places this frequently happens are portions of the skin that are chronically moist because the wetness can disrupt the skin enough to let the bacteria inside. This is one reason why the most common place to find an impetigo rash is around the corners of the mouth, on the chin, or under the nose. Impetigo is also common in places where the skin is irritated or dried out, both of which interfere with the skin's normal barrier function. If the strep is there, or is under a child's fingernails from touching another infected area, scratching introduces the germs to a new spot.

Impetigo has a very characteristic appearance, and you can tell what it is just by looking at it. I have met many experienced parents who are just as good as doctors at recognizing it. It is highly contagious, as are other kinds of strep infections, which is why teachers usually do not want a child with active, untreated impetigo at school. What it looks like is a cluster of crusted, flat, irregularly shaped spots up to a quarter-inch or so in size. The textbook appearance of the crust is honey-colored because it consists of dried tissue-fluid that has oozed out of the infected spot.

An impetigo infection needs to be treated with antibacterial agents. Extensive clusters of sores can be quickly and effectively treated with oral antibiotics. Less-extensive impetigo can be treated with local care and cleaning of the area. You can wash the sores with an antibacterial soap and then put on a thin film of antibiotic ointment, which is available over the counter. If this does not take care of the problem, you can bring your child to the doctor for an antibiotic prescription. Either way, impetigo never requires a nighttime trip to the emergency department.

Strep can cause another fairly common rash, only in this case the strep is not directly infecting the skin but rather is provoking a reaction in the skin. This rash resembles the first variety of rash you read about, red bumps, only in this rash the bumps tend to be very small. The skin often feels like fine sandpaper when you rub it. This rash favors the chest, upper arms, and folds of the skin inside the elbows. The name we give the rash is *scarletina*. It is also called *scarlet fever*, a term that provokes fear, especially in grandparents, because a century ago scarlet fever was a deadly disease. This is no longer so, and we do not understand why that is—perhaps the strep germ changed in some way. But whatever the reason, scarlet fever these days just means a rash with a strep infection, typically of the throat.

There is a another skin problem germs can cause, only this time the germ is usually staph, which you learned about in chapter 9. This germ causes many sorts of infections, some of them serious. It often lives on the skin, where it causes no problems. As with strep, however, if there is a break in the skin, the germ can quickly take advantage, crawl inside, and set up shop. You often see staph as the culprit in infections around a splinter or cut. As we've seen, though, it can invade the skin without an obvious break in the barrier, such as down a hair follicle. When that happens, we call the tender, swollen, and often red result a *boil*.

Staph is notorious for making pus, so it is common for a boil to come to a head and drain. That often is sufficient to cure it, since the body's natural defenses can then take over and clean up the situation. Large, tender boils, however, often need antibiotics to clear them. They also may need to be lanced to let the pus out. Of course both of those possibilities require a trip to the doctor, but as with impetigo, there is no need to do that in the middle of the night.

Although several of the rashes we have discussed so far need medical attention, none of them require a doctor's immediate attention, with the exception of hives complicated by breathing troubles. However, there is one particular rash that needs prompt evaluation because it can be an indication of more-serious problems. This rash has the medical name *petechiae* (pronounced puh-tee-key-eye).

Petechiae are caused by a disruption in the tiny blood vessels in the skin, the capillaries—they break and ooze a little bit of blood into the tissue around them. The result looks like little purple-red blotches, typically only a millimeter or so in size. You cannot feel them, you can only see them.

A few petechiae can be normal, especially following some predictable scenarios. You can give yourself a couple of them if you apply a strong suction to an area of your skin; the suction pops some of the delicate skin vessels. Anything that raises the pressure in the tissue can bring on a few petechiae. For example, if a person has had a strong bout of vomiting, it is common to see petechiae in the face or neck, but especially around the eyes. If you put a tight band around your upper arm, you might see petechiae on your forearm because the back pressure from the band disrupts some of the delicate skin vessels.

The petechiae that are important are caused by a somewhat different mechanism. It still is a problem in the tiny vessels, but it is not because of pressure in the tissues. Rather, it is because the vessels have ruptured on their own. The cause is from a disorder of those tiny blood particles called platelets. Platelets are far smaller than cells. They are bits of cellular dust found throughout the circulation. There are a lot of them, about a billion in each teaspoon of blood.

Platelets have several jobs in the body, one of which is participating in blood clotting. If you do not have a sufficient number of platelets, you will be prone to tiny, spontaneous bleeds in the skin following the disruptions that come from normal wear and tear of the small vessels. A platelet count can be low for one of two reasons: either the body is not making enough platelets, or they are being consumed faster than the body can make them. Serious infections can consume platelets, making them clump, and in the process causing petechiae to form. There are other conditions in children that remove platelets from the circulation and lead to petechiae.

These conditions are not as immediately concerning as those serious infections, but they still need a doctor's evaluation.

If your child's body has petechiae in many places, this does not mean you should necessarily go to the emergency department. But if there are other significant symptoms, particularly fever and lethargy, then you should do that. If your child with petechiae feels well and looks otherwise well to you, the best thing to do is to call your doctor for advice. The odds are high he will want to see your child fairly soon for an evaluation and blood tests, the most important of which is a blood count that includes the platelets.

We have talked about some common causes of rashes in children, but there are hundreds of possible causes. The overwhelming majority of them are not serious. They may cause a child discomfort, but we have ways of relieving those symptoms, and some of them may need a doctor's evaluation at some point. But very few of them call for a trip to the emergency department. Now that you know something of how doctors think about rashes, it is time to turn to our specific scenarios.

WATCHFUL WAITING

Your second-grade daughter has an itchy nose. She has had a bit of a runny nose for several days from a cold, and she has been diligently blowing her nose as she has been taught. But after a few days of this, her nose is red and raw. It itches, so she has been rubbing it frequently. Now you notice that about a half-inch below her nostrils there is a scabby-looking spot that she has picked open several times. When you look closely at the area, you see some amber-colored, crusting spots oriented as satellites around the bigger scab she has been picking at. What is this, and what should you do about it?

What you are looking at are typical impetigo sores. Under the nose is a very common place to see them, another being just outside the lips. There are not very many of them in this case, and most likely you can take care of these at home and then keep an eye on them to make sure they resolve. First wash the area with soap and water. Then put a thin film of antibiotic ointment over the sores. Repeat that at least twice each day until the sores go away. It is important to have your daughter wash her hands frequently to remove any strep germs that are lurking there. Also cut her fingernails short so any scratching she does is less likely to break the skin. If the sores persist or spread, you can call your doctor or bring your daughter in for evaluation.

WATCHFUL WAITING

Your ten-year-old son has come home at the end of a July day spent on a friend's farm. He is dusty and grimy. He also is itching his thighs and upper arms nearly constantly. You see that he has about ten or twenty raised bumps in those areas. The bumps stick up above his skin surface perhaps a quarter-inch or so. Surrounding several of them are red, blotchy areas that form a sort of halo. The ones he can reach have scratches on them from his itching. He otherwise feels fine. What is this and what should you do about it?

This child has typical hives. This case is instructive because much of the time we have no idea what the inciting trigger was. This child has spent a windy day in an environment outside his usual one with multiple potential hive-makers such as grasses and other plants, dusty barns, and animals. The only way to get any clue about what did this is to see if it happens again and then do some detective work. For this episode, the important thing is that he has no swelling in his mouth, difficulty swallowing, or breathing troubles.

If this were your child, you could do a couple of things to make him feel better. First, get him out of his clothes because whatever is inciting the hives could be lurking there. Then wash him off in a bath or shower for the same reason. You can help his itching by giving him some diphenhydramine (Benadryl, many others), which you can get at any pharmacy and most large grocery stores. The medicine will block the histamine that is producing the hives and making him itch. It will also make him drowsy, which at this point in the day is probably a good thing.

CALL THE DOCTOR

We can modify the above scenario just a little to make calling for advice a good plan. Let us say your son has many, many hives. He still has no airway swelling or breathing troubles, but the itching is driving him crazy. You have given him a dose of diphenhydramine, but it does not seem to have helped very much.

In such a situation, it would make sense to call for advice. We have other medications to block the hive process that are more powerful than diphenhydramine. Your doctor may want to consider prescribing one of these, or he may tell you to increase the diphenhydramine dose.

CALL THE DOCTOR

Your one-year-old was diagnosed a few days ago with an ear infection after having fever for a day. He is taking amoxicillin (Amoxil, many others), a commonly prescribed oral antibiotic for this problem. Today he is better. His fever is gone, he is eating normally, and he is acting totally himself. But while putting him to bed you notice his chest and abdomen are covered with tiny red bumps. The rash does not seem to be bothering him at all. For example, he is not itching anywhere. What should you do about this?

The answer to this scenario is that his rash is most likely from the antibiotic. Although almost any medicine can cause a rash, amoxicillin is notorious for doing this. If your son has no other symptoms than the rash, he does not need to be seen by a doctor. However, depending on how far along this child is in his antibiotic course, many doctors would want to change the antibiotic to another one to complete his treatment for the ear infection. The best thing to do in this scenario is to call the doctor to ask for advice.

GO TO THE EMERGENCY DEPARTMENT

Your three-year-old daughter has had upper respiratory infection (URI) symptoms for a week or so, but she has otherwise seemed herself. She has had no fever, and she does not seem to have any aches or pains. Today she has a rash. The rash feels flat on the skin and consists of tiny purple spots—the petechiae you read about earlier. In a few places, the petechiae are merging with each other to make larger purplish splotches. It is early evening on a Friday and you wonder what you should do. Can this wait until Monday, or should you have her evaluated over the weekend?

If this were your child, the best answer to this scenario is you should take her to the emergency department. Your daughter may have a problem with her blood platelets, such as having too few of them circulating in the blood. There are several possibilities for the cause of a low platelet count, but all of them are potentially serious and cannot wait. The doctor can do some simple tests, especially a blood count, to identify the likely problem. Your daughter may need further, more complicated tests to determine what is wrong, and she may need to come into the hospital for treatment.

This child has a not-uncommon condition with the tongue-twisting name of *idiopathic thrombocytopenic purpura*, or ITP for short. Translated into English, each of those words describes the condition: *idiopathic* means we are not sure what causes it; *thrombocytopenic* means low platelet count; and *purpura* is the fancy name for those purple blotches from coalescing petechiae.

The disorder is the result of a child's immune system attacking her platelets and removing them from the circulation. The platelets are sequestered in the spleen, an organ in the upper left part of the abdomen. When you examine a child with ITP, you typically feel the resulting enlarged spleen. We have effective treatment for ITP, and in most children the condition resolves with this treatment, leaving the child healthy again. But it is best to begin this treatment, which generally takes a few days in the hospital, as soon as the disorder is identified.

The URI symptoms in this scenario do not have anything to do with the ITP. I just put those in to remind you that situations are often complicated. It is hard to know sometimes if symptoms are related to each other or are just a coincidence.

GO TO THE EMERGENCY DEPARTMENT

Your eight-year-old daughter has had a fever as high as 104 degrees all afternoon. She has not complained of anything in particular, but she feels a bit weak and dizzy. In the evening you notice she has a rash on her arms and chest. At first the rash looks like small bites—tiny reddish-purple spots. Over the next couple of hours the rash spreads and the spots seem to be getting a little bigger. She still has a temperature of 104 degrees. What should you do about this?

This child's petechial rash is different from that of the child with ITP for a couple of reasons. For one thing, it is progressing much more rapidly. For another, this child is quite ill, with fever and disorientation. That symptom has also progressed quite rapidly. In this case, the petechiae are from a serious, life-threatening bacterial infection. This infection is in the bloodstream, and one of the consequences of the infection is that it consumes platelets. It does many other things too, such as causing the fever and lethargy, but the rash you see is from the destruction of platelets.

This child needs emergency medical attention, which will include blood tests and intravenous antibiotics. She may well need other kinds of therapy as well, depending upon how rapidly the infection is spreading and whether it affects other organs in the body besides the skin, which it nearly always does. Taking your daughter to the emergency department would be the best thing to do in this scenario.

The bacteria that most commonly causes symptoms like these is called *Neisseria meningitidis*, or *meningococcus*. It is contagious. Anyone who has close contact with a documented case should receive oral antibiotics to protect them from contracting the infection. There is also a vaccine that prevents many, although not all, forms of this infection. The American Academy of Pediatrics now recommends that all children receive this vaccine when they are eleven or twelve years old, with a booster vaccination at age sixteen.

CALL 911

In this scenario we modify the story above in a key way. As the rash progresses, becoming more extensive and coalescing into larger purplish blotches, the child's level of consciousness is also changing. She is becoming progressively more lethargic and has spent the last three hours asleep on the couch. When you rouse her she seems incoherent, and you are not sure that she even recognizes you.

This scenario is best handled with a 911 call for help. Things are moving along quickly, and the paramedics will know how to handle the situation. They carry various medications that may be needed to get the child's treatment started.

CHECKLIST AND ACTION PLANS FOR RASHES

The great majority of childhood rashes do not need a trip to the emergency department—most can safely be watched at home. There are a few important exceptions, however, and if you are unsure of what to do, it is a good idea to call your doctor for advice. Since we have discussed several things you can do yourself with some common rashes, this chapter modifies the "Watchful Waiting" category a bit.

Watchful Waiting (and Home Therapy while Watching)

1. Your child appears generally well except for the rash. A mild fever may be present, but not much else.
2. The rash looks like simple impetigo: crusted sores around the mouth and nose. (You may treat this with antibiotic ointment.)
3. The rash looks like simple hives, and your child has no breathing troubles or swelling of the lips or tongue. (You may treat this rash with diphenhydramine [Benadryl, many others].)

Call the Doctor

1. Your child has an impetigo rash that is not improving with home therapy.
2. Your child is taking a new medicine, such as an oral antibiotic.
3. Your child has a progressive diaper rash that is not improving with ordinary lotions and creams.
4. Your child has tender skin boils.

Take Your Child to the Emergency Department

1. Your child has hives accompanied by shortness of breath or swelling around the lips or tongue.
2. Your child has a generalized petechial rash.
3. Besides having the rash, your child appears ill with other symptoms, such as poor oral intake and high fever.

Call 911

1. Your child has hives with severe breathing troubles, such as severe wheezing or severe swelling in and around the mouth or throat.
2. Your child has a petechial rash and is disoriented or otherwise appears severely ill.

11

OVERDOSES, POISONINGS, AND BITES

Small children are prone to eating things they should not. There are several reasons for this. Toddlers explore their world by tasting things and putting them in their mouths. They also observe their parents taking medicines that are stored in bottles in medicine cabinets, and pills can look like enticing candies. Since the advent of childproof caps for medicine bottles, this has been less of a problem, but young children are amazingly adept at still managing to get those bottles open.

Our houses are also filled with things besides medicines that an older child would never find palatable but that look quite tasty to a small child. Cleaning solutions and other materials often come in colorful, exciting-looking bottles and are made in colors that are hard for a toddler to resist. They often look like juice or soft drinks, and when a toddler sees something interesting, tasting it is often the first logical step to the toddler mind. These solutions also have (or should have) difficult-to-open caps, but once again a small child's ingenuity sometimes wins out.

Adults using these materials are not always diligent in putting the caps back on tightly or storing them in a safe place. Every home with small children should have protective latches on cupboards beneath the sink and other storage sites, but kids can get past those too. Garages are a particularly common spot for tasty-appearing but dangerous things to be stored. And sometimes we put toxic materials in containers different from the ones they came in, containers with non-childproof caps.

Besides these numerous man-made hazards, there are also household and outdoor plants that can cause trouble if you eat them. There are not many of these, but if you are camping with your family and your child toddles off into the woods and chews on a handful of bittersweet berries, you can expect to see some problems. Children get bitten too—by insects, spiders, snakes, and pets. Usually these events are uncomfortable though not serious, but not always.

Ingestion of potentially toxic medicines, household supplies, and all manner of objects is a common reason for children to appear in the emergency department. In my career I have seen children consume an astonishing variety of noxious materials, from dishwater to small batteries to quantities of shredded newspaper. Swallowing someone else's medicines is a very common scenario. The possibilities are endless, and we should not forget the host of small objects we have lying about, such as coins and small parts of toys. The great majority of these things cause no lasting problems except perhaps an upset stomach, but some of them are dangerously toxic.

Toddlers eat things they should not eat out of ignorance. Older children and adolescents, however, not infrequently take things deliberately. Often they are experimenting, but sometimes they are trying to harm themselves. Besides legitimate medications, there unfortunately are illicit drugs available nearly everywhere. Parents do the best they can in talking to their children about drugs, but the drugs are out there, and adolescents will encounter them. This includes alcohol.

This chapter will tell you about a variety of common poisonings, bites, and toxic exposures. We cannot be comprehensive, of course, and because of the wide range of possibilities, a textbook of toxicology is several inches thick and weighs several pounds. The Internet has made the subject more accessible, and even doctors use it to look things up because we cannot know everything either. Besides teaching you about specific poisonings, Drs. Google and Bing can tell you about how doctors approach them.

An important concept doctors use for serious poisonings is the principle of the *toxidrome*, a term made of a mashing together the words *toxic* and *syndrome*. What we look for is a bundle of associated symptoms and signs that together indicate a particular category of poisoning. We call this a toxidrome. Once we identify it, we can proceed with treatment even though we are unsure what specific agent the child took. Sometimes we never learn what it was, but we can still know what to do about it. With a few notable exceptions, most poisonings do not have a specific antidote. The most important part of what we do is support the body's organ function while we wait for the effects of the poison, whatever it was, to wear off.

Sometimes the toxic effects are dangerous in themselves, so we do things to reverse the actions of the agent. An example of this is when a toddler gets into her mother's blood-pressure medicine and the overdose drops the child's blood pressure too low. When that happens, we use other medicines to raise the blood pressure back to safe levels until the poisoning wears off.

A few parents, and many more than a few grandparents, might recall seeing someone having their "stomach pumped" if they ate something they should not have eaten. For many years this was the standard treatment, and it is one that makes intuitive sense. After all, if there is something bad in the stomach, it seems logical to get it out.

The stomach pump came in several varieties. In its most common version, it consisted of a long rubber tube with a funnel on the end and a pumping bulb built into the tube. The way it worked was that end of the tube opposite the funnel was pushed through the child's nose and then down into the stomach. That is the natural path for such a tube to take if you just keep pushing. Once the end of the tube was in the stomach, a clear salt-solution was poured down the funnel, sloshed around in the stomach, and then sucked back out by squeezing the pumping bulb. The process was continued until the fluid came back clear.

We rarely do that now. The main reason is that generally by the time the child gets to the emergency department, most of what he has eaten has already left his stomach. There are some exceptions, such as when the child is in the emergency department very quickly and the ingested material is particularly toxic. Another reason we rarely do this now is that stuffing a tube down a child's nose is scary for the child and uncomfortable, so if it does not help much, it is plain cruel to do it. For those uncommon situations in which we do suck out the stomach contents, we still use a flexible tube, but our current suction device is much more efficient than the old-fashioned stomach pump.

There has been another change over the past couple of decades in how we handle poisonings. After pumping stomachs went by the wayside, physicians commonly recommended a more direct way of emptying the stomach—having the patient vomit. This was the standard way of dealing with the issue in my early years of practice. The agent we used to induce vomiting was *syrup of ipecac.*

Ipecac is an oral medicine extracted from a natural plant root. It has been used by physicians for centuries to induce vomiting, dating back to the time when doctors thought making patients vomit when they were ill was just a good thing to do on general principles. Their misguided notion was that a sick person had mysterious toxins inside them that needed to come out before they could heal. Later ipecac came back as a treatment for poisoning. I still meet the occasional parent or grandparent who has tried it. Do not use it; it does not help and may hurt.

There are two main problems with ipecac. One is that the substance is itself toxic. If you give it to a child, some of it inevitably gets absorbed into the bloodstream, where it can cause lethargy and other side effects. This can complicate our efforts to treat the effects of the poison. The other problem is with the vomiting. Although emptying the stomach through vomiting makes intuitive sense, it actually does not work; research has shown you do not get much of the poison out. Also, ipecac-induced vomiting can persist far longer than is desirable. Finally, the vomiting itself can be dangerous, especially if the child is groggy, because some of the stomach contents can get into the child's airway and lungs. The effects of this can be very serious.

Doctors and poison-control experts once recommended that families with small children keep ipecac at home, and some even distributed free doses. If you run across any of these, throw them away. The syrup is no longer manufactured because of all the problems I described above. In addition, if your child swallows something she should not, do not consider doing anything else to make her vomit, such as putting your finger down the back of her throat to gag her.

So these days we rarely do anything to try to get the swallowed poison out of the stomach. However, there is still something we can do to keep the poison from making it out of the stomach and intestines and into the bloodstream: we can try to inactivate it. This requires that the child be in the emergency department soon after eating the toxin, typically within an hour. We do not use the technique all the time, but when we do it can be very helpful.

A material called *activated charcoal* has the ability to bind to a large number of molecules. It is used in many nonmedical chemical applications, such as water purification systems. Charcoal binds to many medicines, and when placed in the stomach and intestines, it can prevent these medicines from getting into the child's system. *Activated* means the charcoal particles have been modified by introducing millions of microscopic pores into the surface. This increases the surface area of the particles many times over, giving it a huge absorptive surface to bind the toxin.

The raw material is a black powder, and no child can swallow that. The way we give charcoal is in the form of a liquid slurry. This makes it a bit easier to get into a child's stomach, but it is still hard to get a toddler to drink the stuff. The mix also contains *sorbitol*, a substance that speeds up transit time through the intestines, moving the charcoal and its bound toxin quickly out of the child's body.

Before we go any further we should discuss the single most important thing for parents to learn in this chapter: How to use Poison Control. This free service has made an enormous difference in dealing with children, and adults too, who have ingested a poison or toxin. It has saved countless lives. Not only parents use Poison Control—physicians rely on it every day.

Poison Control centers began after World War II, a time when nearly half of all accidents to children were poisonings of one sort of another. Many of these children died. The great majority of physicians did not know how to treat any but the most common poisonings. This is completely understandable because the possibilities are so enormous. Doctors needed help, and the concept of an easily accessible information source was born. The idea was to give doctors quick access to experts in treating poisonings, called *toxicologists*.

Even though the centers were started for doctors, later they opened their phone lines to the public. The results have been spectacular, representing a true milestone in public health that few people appreciate. The statistics show that about three-quarters of all poisonings can be handled over the telephone with the information and advice the centers provide, keeping thousands of children out of the emergency department.

As of this writing, there are sixty-one Poison Control centers spread across the country. They all have the same telephone number: 1-800-222-1222. Put it on your refrigerator for everyone in your home, including baby sitters, to see and refer to. If you call that number, you will automatically be directed to a center in your region. As someone who uses it frequently, I can certify that whoever answers the telephone will be calm, cordial, and knowledgeable. That person also has immediate access to a large array of experts on everything from medicines and cleaning solutions to wild plants and fungi to snakebites and scorpion stings.

Now we can get down to our actual cases and see these principles in action. The scenarios in this chapter are different from those in other chapters because, for ingestions and poisonings, every parent has the key resource of Poison Control to call for advice. Just imagine how many emergency department visits would be saved if a similar nation-wide system were in place for other emergency issues occurring at odd hours.

WATCHFUL WAITING

Your child is sick with a fever. You and your husband have been giving him ibuprofen (Motrin, many others) every six hours as your doctor recommended. You gave your child a dose and put him to bed. A half-hour later he is fussing in his room and your husband, unaware you have given him the medicine, gives him another full dose. When the two of you discover what has happened, you are unsure what to do. Could the double dose harm him? Should you call Poison Control about this?

This is actually a common scenario. I have encountered it both under the circumstances above and when parents sort of push the envelope with fever therapy, giving a bit more than the recommended dose with the thought that a little more might help quicker.

That idea is not a good one. The doses you read on a bottle of either ibuprofen or acetaminophen—another fever- and pain-reducing drug available without prescription—are the ones to use. Giving more will not make them work better.

On the other hand, the doses on the bottles are based upon a child's age because that is easier for parents to understand and use. You read about this in chapter 3, but it bears repeating. The doses on the box are actually a bit less than physicians use. The standard dose we use is 10 milligrams per kilogram of body weight. There are 2.2 kilograms per pound. Since ibuprofen liquid is 100 milligrams per teaspoon, that works out to about 1 teaspoon for every 22 pounds that the child weighs.

Taking all this into account, the answer to this scenario is that these parents do not need to do anything because a single double-dose of ibuprofen will not hurt this child. One of the side-effects of ibuprofen, especially if taken chronically for days and days, is an upset stomach. It is possible this child could experience that, at least briefly, but that is unlikely. For all these reasons, these parents can safely observe how this child does at home. They do not need to call Poison Control for advice. If they did, they would be told that simple observation is enough.

CALL THE DOCTOR

Your eighteen-month-old is crawling around in her older brother's room. Like many ten-year-olds' rooms, the place is a mess, with toys scattered across the floor. Among the toys are assorted small components to metal and plastic construction kits. Your older child is deeply engrossed in a construction project and does not pay any attention to his little sister. Like most toddlers, your daughter puts almost any new object in her mouth as part of exploring what it is. She reaches for a small metal strut. This attracts your son's attention, and he sees her put it in her mouth. He goes to take it away, but finds it is gone—she has swallowed it. She does not cough or choke, just gets upset for a minute or so, after which she seems fine. Your son brings her to you after the event. What should you do? Anything?

This is a very common scenario, since small children will deliberately or accidentally swallow almost anything they can put in their mouths. Of course, if a child is choking on whatever she put in her mouth, that can be an emergency. In this case the child shows no distress at all, indicating that the toy probably made it into her stomach.

As a general rule, anything sufficiently small for a child to swallow is small enough to pass all the way through the digestive tract and make it out in the stool. Since this child is a toddler in diapers, it is an easy matter to just watch for that to happen in a day or two. This assumes, however, that the object made it into the stomach, an important distinction. By the way, even though it may seem logical in some ways, for all the reasons you read about earlier in this chapter, you should not try to make the child vomit the object back out.

The reason calling for advice in this situation is the best course is that what to do depends upon several things, most importantly if the object reached the stomach. Sometimes these things hang up at the valve connecting the esophagus, the swallowing tube, with the stomach. This particularly seems to happen with larger coins, such as quarters. Most of the time if an object is stuck at the entry to the stomach, the child will show some signs of discomfort, especially when she swallows. But the lack of such discomfort does not mean the object is not stuck there.

If your child does something like this and is clearly uncomfortable afterward, or if she refuses to drink because it hurts, then you should take her to the emergency department because this suggests the object is lodged at the entry to her stomach. But if, like this child, she looks fine, it is a good idea to call your doctor because how to proceed is a judgment call.

This particular object is metal. That means it will show up on an x-ray. Many physicians will suggest that you take your child in for an x-ray to identify where the object is, but some might advise waiting a while if she continues to appear totally fine.

If the x-ray shows that the object has made it into the stomach, then it is generally safe to just watch for it to pass through over the next couple of days. If, however, the thing is stuck at the entry to the stomach, then it needs to be dealt with. How exactly to do that varies. If it is a coin, emergency department physicians have several tricks they can try to see if they can get the coin to drop into the stomach, after which it will pass downstream. One trick is to have the child drink a carbonated beverage, since the reflex of burping can make the coin drop down. Of course that approach requires waiting an hour or more in the emergency department and then repeating the x-ray. If a child is having discomfort, the sudden disappearance of the discomfort is a good sign that the object has made it to the stomach because when that happens the symptoms go away.

If the object will not pass, or if the x-ray suggests that it will not, then the object needs to be removed. This is done by sedating the child and then passing a long, lighted tube, called an *endoscope*, through the child's mouth and then inserting a special tool down the endoscope to grab the object and pull it out.

As noted, if the x-ray shows that the object has made it into the stomach, then it is usually safe to leave the object alone and wait for it to pass through the digestive tract. I write "usually" because there are some important exceptions to this general principle. One of them is if the object is oddly shaped or sharp, such as an open safety pin or nail (yes, children sometimes swallow these things). This is again a judgment call by the emergency department physician, since circumstances vary.

Another important exception is if the child has swallowed a battery, particularly the kind of small, round batteries that power watches and many other things. Batteries will leak caustic materials that can damage the stomach and intestines, and they need to be taken out quickly. Fortunately batteries can be identified by x-ray. The same endoscopic tools we use to remove objects stuck at the entry to the stomach can be pushed on into the stomach and used to remove objects there. However, they cannot reach things that have moved beyond the stomach.

If your child swallows an object that is not metal, such as a plastic toy, things get a bit more complicated because we often cannot use an x-ray to see the object, although it is surprising how many toys are slightly *radiopaque*, meaning we can make them out on an x-ray, however faintly. In this situation too, it makes sense to call your doctor for advice. If the child shows no symptoms at all, many physicians will advise you to wait and see if the object passes. It is another judgment call.

GO TO THE EMERGENCY DEPARTMENT

Your three-year-old daughter manages to climb up to the medicine cabinet above the bathroom sink and grab a bottle of acetaminophen (Tylenol, many others). Although the bottle has a childproof cap, she gets it open somehow. Your ten-year-old son finds his sister sitting on the floor intently picking up the capsules and eating them. He takes them all away and tells you about it when you get home an hour later.

In spite of eating the capsules, your child looks totally fine. You try to figure out how many she took, but you are not sure how many were in the now half-empty bottle. Your son says he found ten or fifteen on the floor. What should you do? Should you watch her for a few hours to see if she gets sick? Should you take her to the emergency department? If you should, can you drive her there yourself or should you call 911 for an ambulance?

This scenario is another common one. Acetaminophen can be found in millions of medicine cabinets, and those childproof bottle caps are not infallible. In addition, the last user of the bottle does not always snap or screw the top back on completely. Acetaminophen is also part of many nonprescription medicines. If you browse the cold-remedy aisle of any pharmacy and read the labels, you will find that a large number of them have acetaminophen in them because fever and pain are frequent symptoms with colds and flu. These medicines also can cause acetaminophen overdoses in children, especially because they are often sold in tasty (to a toddler) liquid forms. They have childproof caps too, but the screw-on caps can become crusted with dried medicine left over from previous openings, making it difficult to get the cap back on tightly. I have seen several instances of that.

Acetaminophen in the usual doses is quite safe. However, overdoses of this drug can be extremely toxic. Fortunately, the toxicity is not immediate; we have several hours at least to counteract the effects of the drug. The toxicity is also deceptive, in that it does not occur right away. Even many hours after taking an overdose, the person does not feel ill at all. There are no symptoms of any sort.

The toxicity from acetaminophen is not caused by the drug itself. Rather, it comes from components of the drug that appear as the body metabolizes, or breaks down, the medicine. This means that before toxicity appears, the acetaminophen needs to be absorbed into the bloodstream, transported to the liver, and processed there. These dangerous components of the drug do not cause any symptoms either, at least at first. The subsequent symptoms that can potentially occur are from damage to the liver, something that takes many hours or even days to appear. If things progress that far, the situation is very serious, and sometimes there is little we can do.

This delay in toxic damage is fortunate because it gives us time to prevent it. We have a very effective antidote for acetaminophen poisoning. It has the chemical name *n-acetylcysteine*, or *Mucomyst* for short. It works by neutralizing the actions of those breakdown products of the drug before they can do any harm. Mucomyst can be given either by mouth or intravenously. For many years only an oral version of Mucomyst was available, but it has several problems. It smells and tastes terrible—a real problem for getting small children to take it—and it often causes abdominal upset and vomiting. The intravenous version has many fewer unpleasant side-effects, and for that reason it has been used increasingly more frequently over the last several years. The oral version is still available, though.

Receiving the antidote therapy for acetaminophen overdose is not simple. It does not consist of just a dose or two. The oral version requires several days of therapy, while treatment with the intravenous form takes nearly twenty-four hours. This prolonged therapy is necessary to make sure all the toxic components leave the child's system. This means the child needs to come into the hospital to get the therapy.

The key question with acetaminophen overdose is this: How do we know which children need the antidote therapy? For example, does the child in this scenario need it? Fortunately for children and parents, we have excellent guidelines to help us answer the question of who needs to come into the hospital for up to several days of treatment and who can just go home from the emergency department.

The guidelines are to some extent based upon the amount of acetaminophen the child took, although often we are unsure of that. The most important thing is the level of acetaminophen in the child's blood, something we can easily measure. Extensive research has divided the potential for toxicity into three zones: unlikely, possible, and probable. What we need to know is the child's blood level at about four hours after the ingestion. Before that time we will be unsure because the drug may still be being absorbed. So if you bring your child to the emergency department less than four hours after she took the drug, the doctors will want you to wait there until enough time has passed to make the test reliable.

Once we know the four-hour acetaminophen level, we have some idea of the potential for toxicity, but often the child still needs to be observed in the hospital until a second level can be drawn a few hours later. When we have two values, we can use a standardized chart to decide what to do. If the ingestion is a potentially large one, or if the amount is unknown, we often start antidote therapy while waiting to see what the levels are. The antidote can always be stopped if it turns out not to be needed.

Therefore the correct answer to this scenario is that, if this were your child, you should bring her to the emergency department, no matter the hour, to have her blood levels of acetaminophen checked. You should not be surprised if she is admitted to the hospital while the doctors are figuring out if she needs a complete course of therapy. Since children like this one are completely well shortly after taking the acetaminophen, there is no reason to call an ambulance. Parents of a child in this situation can certainly call Poison Control for advice, but they will be told to bring their child to the emergency department. It is also helpful to bring the medicine bottle and to try to estimate how many pills or capsules the child took.

This is a good time to note that although acetaminophen is a common ingestion, children also still take overdoses of aspirin or aspirin-containing products. Before acetaminophen was available, this was much more common, but it still occurs not infrequently. Aspirin overdose is handled in a similar way to acetaminophen overdose in that we base what we do on a blood level. So if your child has taken too much aspirin, the thing to do again is to bring her to the emergency department for a blood test. If you are unsure if the amount she took is toxic, you can call Poison Control for advice.

CALL 911

Your family is doing its annual cleaning of the garage. In the bustle of hauling out a year's accumulation of junk, nobody notices, until it is too late, that your two-year-old has been drinking from a jug of windshield washer fluid. As with the scenario above, it is mysterious how he got the childproof cap off—perhaps it was not screwed on all the way—but such things happen. He gets your attention when he starts to cough and sputter, after which he seems to be breathing faster than usual. You are not sure how much he drank. What should you do? Do you need to bring him to the emergency department? If so, how?

If this were your child, the answer to this scenario is that you should call for immediate help because the possibility of serious problems is high and those problems can develop very quickly. If you live close to an emergency department, you might bring the child yourself, but the safest thing to do would be to call 911. If you were to call Poison Control about a scenario like this, you would be told to get your child to the emergency department quickly.

Products like windshield washer fluid have several ways they can be toxic to children. The specific components of all these products vary, so it is a good idea to bring along the bottle that lists the ingredients. The number of toxic substances found in garages and basements is huge: cleaning solutions, weed killers, fertilizers, and many more. I chose windshield washer fluid because it comes in such an attractive blue color, and it is generally in a transparent bottle. It also tastes sweet to toddlers at first sip.

Compounds like windshield washer fluid can cause trouble in several ways. The most immediate of these is breathing troubles if the child gets even a few teaspoons or so into his lungs. This can happen in a couple of ways. A child who takes a big swallow of windshield washer fluid often sputters because, after that first sip, the fluid does not taste very good. When he sputters, a bit of the fluid can easily get into his lungs. Another way is if the child spontaneously vomits after swallowing several gulps. On the way back out, some of the fluid can easily go down the wrong way and into the windpipe.

When solvents like windshield washer fluid reach the lungs, they can cause quite a bit of damage. The first sign of a problem, after the coughing, is rapid breathing. What happens next is that the lungs begin to get soggy, with fluid oozing into the airspaces. If and when things worsen, and that can happen quickly, the child can develop a need for extra oxygen. One good reason to call for help is that paramedics bring oxygen and other airway supplies with them and know how to use them. Depending on how severe the lung injury is, the child can become very ill indeed, requiring much more than just some oxygen. He may need intensive care and, in the worst cases, the help of a breathing machine. So any kind of solvent inhalation, even a little bit, can cause severe problems.

Even if the child does not get any of the substance into his lungs, windshield washer fluid and many other similar products found in the garage are toxic if swallowed. They often contain *methanol*, an alcohol that also goes by the common name of *wood alcohol*. Methanol is extremely toxic, as many unfortunate people discovered during Prohibition when methanol was sometimes used to adulterate illicit moonshine. It is a close cousin of *ethanol*, the alcohol found in beer, wine, and liquor, but methanol produces very different toxic effects on the body.

The toxic effects of methanol are potentially very severe. It causes the blood sugar to drop to dangerous levels. It can damage the brain, the eyes, the kidneys, and other organs. It leads to a dangerous accumulation of acid in the blood. It is very evil stuff for a toddler to drink, and it does not take much to cause trouble. As little as two teaspoons of pure methanol can be fatal in the average-size toddler if not treated. The amount of methanol in windshield washer fluid varies, but it is typically 25 to 50 percent or more.

Fortunately, unlike the potential breathing troubles, the toxic effects of methanol on the rest of the body usually take a few hours to develop, and we have an antidote for the poison. But this antidote needs to be started as soon as possible, and of course the more methanol the child has ingested, the quicker the toxic effects appear. Treatment of methanol poisoning generally means admission to a pediatric intensive care unit because doctors have to be ready to handle all the potential complications.

Besides methanol, there are other quite toxic solvents often found in garages, basements, and work sheds. Kerosene is another example of something that can cause immediate and serious breathing troubles. Turpentine, paint thinner, and paint-stripping agents are also toxic. If your child gets into any of these, you should take him to the emergency department because even small quantities of many of these agents can be toxic. If he is in any distress at all with his breathing, call 911. As always, if you are unsure what to do, you can call Poison Control, but they will undoubtedly tell you the same thing.

CHECKLIST AND ACTION PLANS FOR OVERDOSES, POISONINGS, AND BITES

All of the action plans in this chapter use calling Poison Control as a default if you are unsure what to do. Poison Control is uniformly helpful and takes all questions seriously. You should never hesitate to call because, for example, you think your question is silly or you worry you will be criticized for not supervising your child sufficiently. On the other hand, Poison Control is not the public library or a substitute for an Internet search engine when you just want information. They are there to offer specific advice when your child has gotten into something he should not have. If you are unsure what to do and your child has taken a household product, there also should be advice on the box or bottle. Remember that Poison Control can also help you if your child has eaten a plant or been bitten by a snake or other animal.

Watchful Waiting

1. Your child has received as much as two to three times too much of a medicine he is taking already, and he looks fine.
2. Your child has eaten a modest amount of something you are sure is nontoxic from reading the contents, such as shampoo, toothpaste, or crayons.
3. Your child has swallowed an object smaller than the diameter of a nickel and appears fine.

Call Poison Control

1. Your child has taken any medicine not intended for her.
2. Your child has taken a household product and you cannot determine from the label what to do, or the label tells you to call for advice.
3. Your child has eaten a significant amount (more than a bite or two) of a household plant.

Call the Doctor

1. Your child has eaten an object larger than the diameter of a nickel but looks fine.

2. You have called Poison Control but have problems understanding what they want you to do and why. (This can happen sometimes.)

Go to the Emergency Department

1. You have called Poison Control and they have recommended you go to the emergency department.
2. Your child has swallowed an object and appears uncomfortable afterward.
3. Your child has been bitten by a snake or spider, and you are unsure if it was a poisonous one; or your child has been bitten by a scorpion, another known poisonous animal, or a dog whose vaccination status is unknown.
4. Your child has eaten something and is not acting normally afterward.

Call 911

1. Your child has taken something and afterward has trouble breathing.
2. Your child has taken something and afterward is lethargic.
3. Your child has taken anything containing methanol, lye, paint thinner, turpentine, kerosene, or another caustic material.

12

HEADACHES, CONVULSIONS, AND ALTERED MENTAL STATES

You read about what to do for head injuries in chapter 7. This chapter is about the other brain problems and troubles children may have that do not involve trauma. These are common reasons for parents to bring their child to the emergency department. It is easy to see why, since anything involving the brain is potentially scary.

Before we get into specific problems, recall from chapter 7 some key points of the anatomy of the head. Most of the space inside the skull is taken up by the brain. The brain is covered by several layers of membranes, together called the meninges. The inner membranes are tight against the brain. They are very delicate structures. In contrast, the outer layer, the dura, is a tough, fibrous sheath. The meninges encase the brain and spinal cord, extending all the way down the inside of the spinal column to its base above the hips. Between the layers is a fluid compartment called the subdural space. This space is filled with cerebrospinal fluid. Outside the dura is the skull, and outside that are several layers of muscles before we reach the skin and hair.

The lower part of the front of the head, below the eyes, is composed of structures that are not brain. If you approach the brain from that direction, you have to go deep inside before you reach it.

A couple of components of the front of the head that are important for headaches are the eyes and the sinuses. As you will recall, the sinuses are air-filled cavities. The largest of these are the maxillary sinuses, just below the eyes and above the cheeks. Infants and very small children have only rudimentary sinuses because the sinuses appear and grow as we grow. In fact, by the time we enter primary school, our brain is mostly done growing; the great majority of later increase in head size comes from things that are not brain.

By far the most common problem with the head is when it hurts—a headache. The vast majority of headaches are passing annoyances, but a few have serious, even life-threatening causes. Often a headache is accompanied by other symptoms, such as a sore throat, topics we have touched upon in other chapters. In this chapter we will talk about situations in which the headache is either the only symptom or the most prominent one.

The best way to understand headaches, and thus what to do about them if your child has one in the middle of the night, is to classify them as doctors do. We have several criteria for doing that. Learning about this will also be very helpful to you if you need to call the doctor and describe over the telephone what your child is experiencing. Once you have read about how we classify headaches, you can then understand what these categories mean about the cause of the pain.

The first thing to notice is the location of the headache. The major point here is determining if the pain is localized to one spot, such as being on only one side of the head or behind the eyes or diffusely spread across the skull. Another key point is the quality of the headache. This information can be difficult or impossible to obtain from a child who can only tell you that his head hurts, but it is well worth trying to figure this out because it affects how we approach the problem. One aspect of headache quality is some assessment of how bad it is, how severe the pain. You can get a measure of that simply by looking at what your child is doing. Is he continuing to do his usual activities, is he lying still and refusing to do anything, or is he somewhere in between those extremes? Is the pain a throbbing, pulsatile sort of pain, like a man inside the head whacking rhythmically with a hammer, or is the pain constant, steady? Does anything improve the pain or make it worse? Another consideration is if there are any other symptoms associated with the pain. The presence of nausea or vomiting is a key one. Also important is if the child has a fever or rash.

The timing of the headache also is useful in figuring out the cause. What was the child doing when the headache appeared? Did it appear first thing in the morning? Did it awaken the child from sleep? Probably the most important consideration regarding timing is whether the headache is acute, brand-new, and out of the blue or rather a worsening of a chronic problem. That is, if the child has had headaches like this before, how severe were they and how often did they occur?

Headache is an entirely subjective experience, and many children will not be able to help much by giving specific information. But anything a parent can glean from their child is very useful in deciding what to do. The parent is in the best position to obtain this sort of insight since they know their child well.

By far the most common form of headache, both in adults and children, is what we term a *tension headache*. These have some typical aspects that parents can use to decide what to do. Tension headaches come from things going on in the tissues of the head but outside the skull. That means the brain itself is not involved. The muscles of the head, outside the skull, are quite powerful; when they are tense, the entire head hurts.

A typical tension headache is a steady, squeezing sort of pain. The pain is mild to moderate. It is generally not well localized, although some people will feel it worst behind both eyes. Generally a tension headache will not wake up a child from sleep. There are no associated symptoms, particularly no vomiting. Often it is a recurring problem, frequently associated with things that cause the child stress. Tension headaches can be treated with simple over-the-counter painkillers, such as ibuprofen (Motrin, many others) or acetaminophen (Tylenol, many others). The most important distinction is that tension headaches are not associated with anything being wrong with the brain.

After tension headaches, the second-largest category of headache is *migraine*. This is a catch-all term for headaches that are caused by changes in the blood vessels inside the brain. These blood vessels may dilate, and the resulting increased pressure inside the closed box of the skull makes the head hurt. A migraine headache is characteristically (although not always) pulsatile, meaning it throbs, because as the heart beats, the amount of blood inside the skull goes up and down with the rhythm. Migraine is often localized to one side of the head (or behind one eye) because these blood-vessel changes may not be happening everywhere in the brain.

Migraine also may be associated with nerve symptoms, such as visual disturbances or numbness. These symptoms occur at the beginning of the headache and pass on their own. They are caused by the brain's blood vessels first constricting before they dilate. Abdominal complaints, especially nausea and vomiting, are extremely common with migraine headache. This phenomenon may relate to the strong association between migraine and a tendency to motion sickness. Migraine headaches also often run in families.

Unless it is their first one, of course, people with migraine have had one before, so they often know what it is. But with children it can be hard to tell what is going on. It can be difficult to know if this is a previous headache form or some new variety. So good clues that a headache is a migraine are nausea, vomiting, and visual disturbances such as seeing spots or finding light painful to the eyes.

Migraines do resolve on their own, but that can take hours or sometimes even days, and meanwhile the patient is miserable. Milder migraines can be treated with over-the-counter pain medications, but more severe ones are best treated with other medicines. There is a long list of medications doctors use to treat migraines, and what works for one patient may not work for another. Many people with migraine have certain things, such as foods or activities, that tend to trigger a headache, but for others the occurrences seem random.

The next category of headaches we will talk about are those caused by increased pressure inside the skull. There are several reasons this might happen, most of them serious. Examples are tumors or bleeding inside the skull. These things are rare, but they are what all parents fear. Even though the overwhelming majority of children with headaches have nothing seriously wrong with them, lurking among the thousands of innocent headaches are a few that are not. How can a parent tell when this might be a possibility, and therefore when they should bring their child to the doctor?

The answer is that although there are no hard-and-fast rules, several things can give doctors concern for serious causes. One of these is a persistent, even relentless quality to the headache, such as being present day after day. Another thing to consider is severity. Suspicious headaches are bad ones, and they tend to get progressively worse. They often prevent the child from doing her usual activities. They tend to be worse in the early morning, and often they will awaken a child from a sound sleep. Contrast that with a tension headache, for which a nap often improves the symptoms. Finally, headaches from something seriously abnormal inside the skull often cause persistent vomiting, especially in the morning.

A last serious headache cause is the pain that comes from inflammation of the meninges, that system of membranes covering the brain and spinal cord. The condition is called *meningitis*. In children, nearly all of these situations are caused by infection, either by a virus or a bacterial germ. The viral causes, with a few rare exceptions, are milder and pass without treatment. In contrast, meningitis from bacteria is an emergency that needs prompt antibiotic therapy. Bacterial meningitis is now less common since we have a good vaccine (HIB) to prevent the variety that was once the most common, called *Haemophilus influenza*. The other two varieties of bacterial meningitis also have vaccines that help prevent them, but these vaccines are not nearly as effective as HIB. We still see cases.

The headache from meningitis is severe. Most important, however, are the things that go along with the headache: high fever, a stiff neck, confusion or lethargy, and sometimes a rash. You read an example of this last situation in the final scenario in chapter 10.

The range of what to do if your child has a headache thus ranges from nothing—that is, do not worry about it—to calling for an ambulance. That is a disturbingly wide range of possibilities. Still, there are commonsense rules a parent can use. If your child has had headaches before but is having a more severe version of her usual one, that can wait until morning at least. So can a more severe headache if the child is alert. Remember, other than meningitis, headache is largely a chronic problem. Unless it is head-splittingly severe, if the child is otherwise himself, it can wait. The key exception, which leads us to our next topic, is changes in what doctors call *level of consciousness*.

This term refers to your degree of alertness and willingness to interact with the world around you. A rough-and-ready assessment of this that has been used for many years is if the person knows who they are, where they are, and what day it is. We also have fancier evaluation scales for doing this assessment, including one that we use particularly to assess patients who have a lower level of awareness. You may hear terms like *stupor* and *coma*, but there are no exact definitions of those terms.

Broadly speaking, when a doctor assesses a change in a child's level of consciousness, he sorts the change into one of several broad categories: mild, moderate, or severe. Examples of a mild alteration in level of consciousness are a child who is disoriented, not acting normally for himself, or unable to recognize his parents. Such children may be dozing but are easily aroused.

A child with a moderate change in level of consciousness appears to be in a sleep from which she cannot be aroused by touching her, although she will respond to something like pinching her finger by withdrawing her hand. A child with a severe change in level of consciousness does not respond to stimuli of any sort. Children this deeply unreactive to their surroundings often have abnormal breathing patterns.

What should a parent do if their child is experiencing any of these symptoms? Altered mental states mean something is amiss in the brain. Unless the problem is fleeting and mild, children experiencing these symptoms should be promptly evaluated in the emergency department. The possibilities for what is wrong are many, but they all need a doctor's evaluation, and often tests, to figure out what is wrong. A possible exception is a child who has a high fever, say over 104 degrees, and who seems confused and not himself when the fever is high, but who promptly becomes mentally normal again when the fever comes down after a dose of ibuprofen or acetaminophen. This is not uncommon.

There is another important category of altered consciousness that concerns children under the age of six months or so, most typically between two and three months. These are situations in which the child becomes limp and unresponsive, usually quite suddenly. These events are ones in which an observer, most often a parent, believes from what she sees that something serious has happened. An expert committee defined these spells some years ago as episodes that are frightening to the observer and characterized by some combination of *apnea* (a pause in breathing), color change (usually to dusky or pallid but occasionally flushed), marked change in muscle tone (usually severe limpness), choking, and gagging. In some cases, the observer fears that the infant has died. The official name for these occurrences is *apparent life-threatening event*, or ALTE for short.

There are many potential causes for an ALTE, some of them serious. Over half of them turn out to be nothing, but from a parent's perspective, this is a decision best made by a doctor. ALTEs are not rare; large studies show that between 0.5 to 1 percent of all children will have one. We should not be surprised by this, since identifying an ALTE is subjective; what is concerning for one parent may not be for another.

The best thing to do if you believe your child has had such an episode is to trust your judgment that something might be wrong and to bring him to the doctor. Most of the time this will mean a visit to the emergency department. The doctors there are all well-versed in how to handle these situations. Most of the time that means an admission to the hospital for tests and skilled observation to see if the ALTE happens again. The good news is that the majority of these events turn out to be benign. But no parent should take the chance of ignoring something serious.

What sorts of things can cause an ALTE? Bear in mind that for just over half we have no explanation. For the rest, around a quarter stem from problems in the gastrointestinal tract, particularly regurgitation, or reflux, of stomach contents. Infants have a reflex in which they often respond to food coming up the wrong way by pausing in their breathing. About an eighth or so of ALTEs are from problems in the nervous system, such as a convulsion, what doctors call a *seizure*. Around a tenth are from respiratory infections; infants also have a reflex that can make them respond to infection by abnormal breathing patterns. These three causes account for well over 90 percent of the ALTEs for which a cause is identified; the remaining ALTEs are caused by a long list of rarer conditions. But remember, for half of the children we have no explanation.

Seizures can cause other forms of altered mental states besides an ALTE, so this is a good time to discuss what causes them. The brain runs on electricity. It is composed of billions of interconnected cells that communicate with each other using electrical currents, which they generate using chemical reactions inside the cells. Doctors learned many decades ago that these electrical currents between the cells on the surface of the brain can be observed and measured using the very simple technique of placing a series of electrodes on the scalp. The test is called an *electroencephalogram*, or EEG. It is really a very simple test and does not hurt at all. When the fine wires from the electrodes are connected to the main unit, it displays the pattern of the brain waves, the electrical signals, on a screen. This pattern is normally very organized and regulated, and neurologists identified many years ago which patterns are normal and which are not.

A seizure is the result of all the wiring connections on the surface of the brain, the *cortex*, becoming deranged. Instead of the brain cells conversing back and forth, waiting their turn to speak in an organized manner, all the cells fire off their electrical signals at once. This problem may involve part of the brain surface or all of it. When most or all the brain cells misfire in this chaotic manner, the person loses consciousness because orderly communication between cortex brain cells is necessary for awareness. A person with a seizure often shows abnormal eye movements and twitching of the arms and legs. This comes from the disorganized electrical signals in the brain stimulating the muscles.

There are several kinds of seizures. A *generalized seizure* involves the entire brain, and the child usually loses consciousness. Typically there is jerking of the arms and legs, but not always—sometimes there is just a sudden loss of consciousness. Seizures can also involve only part of the brain. These may manifest themselves as a child's sudden loss of awareness of his surroundings, with or without unusual movements such as twitching of the eyes or facial muscles.

It is a scary thing for a parent to see her child have a seizure, and to non-physicians it appears to be a dangerous thing in itself. Sometimes this is so, but the most common form of seizure in children generally passes within a few minutes and causes no long-standing harm to the child. But it is a potentially serious event. A seizure is a sign that the surface of the brain is being irritated by something. It requires at least a doctor's advice, and often an evaluation, even in the middle of the night, because the most important thing to find out is the underlying reason for the seizure. An exception to this general principle would be if your child already has a known seizure problem and perhaps takes medicine for it, and from experience with the problem and advice from your doctor you know what to do if he has one.

As noted earlier, by far the most common cause of seizures in young children is what we call a *febrile seizure*. One to three percent of all children will have at least one of them. They occur mostly in toddlers and follow a rapid rise in temperature. What is important is not how high the fever gets, but how fast it rises. A typical scenario for a child with a febrile seizure is that his temperature goes from normal to over 102 degrees in an hour or so. These seizures usually last less than five minutes and resolve on their own. They tend to run in families and are more common in boys than girls. A child who has one is more likely to have another, but having more than three or four during the toddler years is uncommon.

Before we get into specific scenarios, you should learn something about the common tests doctors use to evaluate severe headaches, altered mental status, and seizures. You just read about the EEG test. We also use CT and MRI scans to get images of the brain, tests you read about in chapter 7. But many times we do not need these sophisticated tests of the brain to determine what the problem is. Even today, as was the case many decades ago, the most important aspect of any evaluation is a conversation with the parents and an examination of the child.

There is another key test in evaluating headaches, seizures, and alterations in mental status: the lumbar puncture, or spinal tap. As you also read in chapter 7, the brain essentially floats in a tank of fluid, called cerebrospinal fluid, or CSF. This fluid acts a kind of shock absorber for milder blows to the head. The fluid is part of a dynamic system. The brain is actually hollow, with CSF-filled cavities in the center. New fluid is constantly being made in these cavities. From there it circulates out of the middle of the brain through a series of channels. Once out, it bathes the outer surface of the brain, where special structures absorb the fluid into the bloodstream. This one-way cycle of CSF involves a lot of fluid; the average adult makes about a quart a day.

A key aspect of how CSF circulates is that a portion of the fluid goes down from the brain and fills up the space surrounding the spinal cord. Even though the spinal cord ends at about the middle of the back, the fluid-filled cavity it floats in extends all the way down to the tailbone. This means we can place a needle in the lower part of the space, below where the spinal cord ends, and easily get a sample of CSF. The important point is that this CSF came from the brain, so a sample of fluid from the lower back can tell us what is happening up in the brain. This procedure of sampling that CSF is called a lumbar puncture, or spinal tap. The spinal tap is an important diagnostic tool for emergency department physicians. What do we use it for?

Recall that the surface of the brain is covered with delicate membranes collectively called the meninges. These membranes are not uncommonly infected in children, a condition called meningitis. When the meninges are inflamed from infection, cells leak out into the CSF that are not there normally. A spinal tap allows us to check for this—it is a crucial test for discovering if meningitis is present.

The brain is a complicated and fascinating organ. More than any of the others, it is what makes us uniquely human. Now it is time to get to scenarios involving the brain that put into action the principles you have read about.

WATCHFUL WAITING

Your twelve-year-old daughter has been getting headaches over the past several months. At first it was just every week or so, but now she has them nearly every day in the late afternoon. This evening she has a particularly bad one, the worst so far. She even vomits a few times at the beginning of the headache. She is well otherwise— no fever, cough, or other symptoms—and she is alert. You are understandably worried about these headaches and you wonder if you should bring her in to the emergency department to see a doctor tonight. Should you?

This scenario is a common one for migraine headaches. When you talk to a child with symptoms like these, you may get the story that the headache is mostly in one part or another of the head, or may have begun in one region and then become general over the head. But children do not keep such close tabs on their symptoms as adults do, so more likely you will just hear from her that her head hurts. Another aspect of this scenario that is typical for migraine is the vomiting, particularly at the onset of the headache.

There are a few other details that are important in this story. One is the chronicity of the symptoms. Although your daughter has a severe headache, it consists of a worse version of those that she has had before. This indicates it is not a new process, but rather an exacerbation of problems she has had for several months. Another point is that the child, although in pain, is alert and oriented. If she were not, then this would become the most important aspect of the scenario.

Taking all these things into consideration, it would be perfectly fine for you to observe this child at home, perhaps giving her a dose of ibuprofen or acetaminophen for the pain. Considering that this has been an ongoing problem, though, it would be a good idea for you to bring her to the doctor sometime soon for an evaluation.

There is another aspect of this story that is important: the nature of the vomiting. In this scenario it happened a few times at the beginning of the headache. Headaches from other causes, particularly increasing pressure inside the skull, also often cause vomiting. The differences are the severity and timing of the vomiting. If the vomiting is persistent and severe, and especially if it occurs first thing in the morning, it should prompt a call to your physician. This is a good time to remind you that if you are unsure or nervous about what to do, the best approach is to bump your action plan up to the next category.

CALL THE DOCTOR

Your three-year-old son has had a runny nose for a day or two. This afternoon you put him down for a nap. About an hour later you hear an odd noise coming from his room and you go in to check on him. You find him lying on his back in his crib. He is flushed and sweating. He is making jerking motions with his arms and legs. Before you can do anything, the movements stop. Afterward he appears drowsy for a couple of minutes, but after that he is alert. He is crying and upset, and you take his temperature—it is 102 degrees. You give him some ibuprofen, and within forty-five minutes his temperature is normal. He even looks now to be his usual, active self. What should you do?

Your son has undoubtedly had a febrile seizure. As you read earlier, the characteristics of these are that they are generalized—

meaning they involve the entire body—and brief, less than five minutes in duration. They also typically occur following a rapid rise in temperature, such as this child experienced.

How we handle first febrile seizures has undergone an evolution over the past decades. Three decades ago, doctors typically performed an extensive evaluation, including an EEG and often a spinal tap. What they were looking for was an underlying seizure disorder, such as epilepsy, or an infection around the brain, such as meningitis. Since then we have come to realize that the vast majority of children with stories like this do not have either of those serious problems. Of course there are important qualifications to consider here. The most important is that afterward the child seemed himself, especially after his fever came down.

There is also the question of where the fever is coming from. This child has had upper respiratory tract infection (URI) symptoms for several days, although he has not had any fever with his runny nose and congestion. Usually when a child has a fever from a URI, it comes early in the illness. In this scenario, the odds are better than even that the fever is from an ear infection. As you read in chapter 4, it is common for these infections to follow several days of URI symptoms. So how should the parent of a child like this approach the situation?

The first issue is the seizure. You have read that brief febrile seizures are common and lead to no long-standing problems. But that is not really a determination parents should make without help. Sometimes a seizure has other characteristics that make it more concerning. One is involvement of only a part of the body. Another is a seizure lasting longer than just a couple of minutes. Or it may be not a single seizure but a flurry of short seizures with pauses in between. At other times a parent may be unsure if their child really has returned to his normal baseline level of consciousness afterward. In fact, some lethargy after any seizure, febrile seizures included, is common. It is a judgment call if a particular child's grogginess after a seizure is within the expected range or not.

For these reasons, in a scenario like this it is best for the parent at least to call the doctor for advice. If your own particular situation means that you do not have ready access to that kind of advice, then a trip to the emergency department is a perfectly reasonable thing to do.

As you read in chapter 3, fever alone is not a reason to bring your child to the emergency department. Even if the child in this scenario has an ear infection, something we often treat with antibiotics, it is not an emergency and can wait at least until morning. This is something else that a call to the doctor for advice could help you sort out.

Besides calling the doctor, another useful thing to do in a scenario like this is to continue to use medicine for the child's fever on a scheduled basis because another sudden rise in temperature might provoke another seizure. The instructions on a bottle of ibuprofen or acetaminophen will tell you how frequently you can give your child the medicine.

GO TO THE EMERGENCY DEPARTMENT

It is dinnertime but your fourteen-year-old son has not come down from his bedroom. He came home from school saying he felt a bit ill and would lie down for a nap. You go up to get him and find him asleep in his bed. When you talk to him he rouses a little bit but is still quite drowsy. You snap on the lights to get a better look at him, and he wants you to turn the lights off again because they hurt his eyes. He says he has a headache, and his neck hurts too. This is unusual for him; he rarely has headaches. You feel his forehead and it feels warm. Your thermometer confirms he has a temperature of 102 degrees. He says the headache has been getting worse over the past couple of hours, and he says he has had very little or nothing to drink all day. What should you do? Should you give him medicine for his fever and headache and then see how he is in the morning? Or does he need to see a doctor tonight?

This scenario is concerning for several reasons. Your son has a severe headache, but he rarely has headaches at all. He is drowsy, even a bit disoriented. Besides the headache, he says his neck hurts. He has not had anything to drink all day, and he is therefore undoubtedly somewhat dehydrated. All of these things suggest a good possibility that he has meningitis. If he does not, this story would be enough for most physicians to suggest a spinal tap to answer the question. If this were your child, you would be right to be worried, but realize that the vast majority of children with meningitis recover completely. However, it does require prompt evaluation since delay could potentially make things worse. For all of these reasons, the best course of action would be to bring him to the emergency department.

CALL 911

Your sixteen-year-old daughter has been in her usual state of good health until today. Suddenly, during lunch, she slumps to the floor after making a strange cry. She then proceeds to have a several minutes of shaking of her arms and legs. Her lips also become a bit dusky-colored, and she drools some saliva from the corner of her mouth. Afterward she remains on the floor. She moans a little when you shake her but otherwise does not respond to you. What should you do?

This child has had a serious event, what we call a *grand mal seizure*. At this point there is no way to tell the reason for her seizure, although there are several possibilities. She needs to see a doctor to figure things out. If this were your child, the best way to get her medical attention quickly would be to call 911. For one thing, in her current state you could not get her to the emergency department yourself. For another, a seizure like this is often fol-lowed by another one. The paramedics will have medicines to inter-rupt any further seizures.

Sometimes people who have seizures have blockage of their airway, either during the seizure or afterward. The best way to keep your daughter's airway clear is to reposition her. So while you are waiting for the paramedics to arrive, it is a good idea to turn her on her side to keep the tongue and soft tissues of the back of her throat from obstructing her airway.

CHECKLIST AND ACTION PLANS FOR HEADACHES, CONVULSIONS, AND ALTERED MENTAL STATES

The brain and the rest of the nervous system are complicated, and the possibilities for your child's nervous system making *you* ner-vous are wide-ranging. You read about how to approach head inju-ries in chapter 7. This chapter covers what to do with problems not related to trauma. As a general rule, isolated headaches rarely re-quire a trip to the emergency department. Altered mental states often do, and convulsions usually do. As with the checklists for previous chapters, it is a good idea to move your action plan to the next-most-serious category if you are unsure what to do. Problems with the brain can be scary, but any parent can still use a simple, systematic approach that is similar to how doctors approach these issues. One thing to keep in mind is that poisoning, the ingestion of something toxic, may manifest as altered mental status. Toddlers take things by accident; sometimes older children do so deliberate-ly. So we always consider that possibility.

Watchful Waiting

1. Your child's headache is mild to moderate—only minimally affecting her usual activities or state of alertness.
2. Your child has had headaches like this in the past.
3. The headache is not accompanied by other symptoms.

Call the Doctor

1. Your child's headaches have been frequent and persistent.
2. Your child has a headache accompanied by severe vomiting, high fever, or a rash.
3. Your child has a brief—a minute or two—spell of altered awareness, but seems fine now. (This may be reported to you by his teacher.)

Go to the Emergency Department

1. Your child has a severe headache with high fever, stiff neck, or rash.
2. Your child has persistent altered mental status, with or without other symptoms.
3. Your child has experienced what looks to you to be a convulsion, but it has now stopped, and she is breathing normally.
4. Your infant has experienced what looks to you to be an ALTE—some combination of a pause in breathing, color change, and marked limpness—but now he looks normal.

Call 911

1. Your child is unconscious—unresponsive to you.
2. Your child is experiencing what looks to you to be a convulsion, and it is continuing longer than several minutes.

3. Your child is having breathing troubles during or following what appears to you to be a convulsion or an ALTE.

13

ALLERGIC REACTIONS

Allergies seem to wax and wane as an explanation for troublesome symptoms in children. This is not a new phenomenon. Allergies have a long history of being invoked as a cause of symptoms that are otherwise difficult to explain. For example, those of you who have seen the wonderful 1930s Disney production of *Pinocchio* will recall that the sly fox diagnoses the hero's conflicted feelings as evidence of allergies. In that era allergies were all the rage as an explanation for unusual symptoms. Now, eighty years after that movie, I still hear "allergies" as an all-purpose answer (and sometimes dodge) to explain mysterious symptoms. This should tell you there is a lot of loose description and confusion out there regarding exactly what is and is not an allergy. In some ways, "allergies" can be a sort of hand-waving non-explanation for many things.

This chapter will tell you exactly what allergies are—what they explain and what they cannot explain. Once in a while allergic reactions require an evaluation in the emergency department. This is uncommon, but it happens. But before you can understand which allergic reactions might require a trip to the emergency department, you need to understand what an allergy is. Non-physicians often use the term to describe any intolerance to something. To a physician, however, *allergy* means a very specific thing.

True allergic reactions are caused by specialized components of the immune system. Immunity is what allows our bodies to fight infections. It has several major pathways. One of them involves *antibodies*, which are protein molecules that circulate in our bloodstream. Antibodies are highly specific; they recognize only a single thing, such as a germ. They circulate throughout the body, on the lookout for their particular target. When they find it, they bind to the enemy like a key in its lock, marking it for other components of the immune system to kill.

This intricate arrangement requires that the body have previously encountered the germ so that the body can produce a stock of antibodies that know their target. When the immune system meets any new foreign material that enters the body, such as a germ, it first sniffs the intruder over. It then uses the foreign material as a template to teach specialized factory cells how to make antibodies that will recognize the germ if they see it again.

A good example of how this process works is vaccination. The reason children today are immune from so many infectious scourges of the past is that scientists have constructed vaccines to prevent it. These consist of what are inactive pieces of a particular germ. By themselves these materials cause no disease; they are made up of those portions of the naturally-occurring germ normally used by the immune system to raise antibodies against it. So when a child receives the vaccine, his body makes antibodies that will protect him from that microbe in the future without having seen the actual, fully intact germ before.

The circulating population of specific antibodies does fade out over time, although the speed and degree to which this happens depends on several things, such as the particular vaccine and the age of the person. That is why many vaccines require a booster shot or two some years later to remind the immune system. Most vaccines also require an initial series of several shots, rather than a single one, to rev up the immune response to reach long-lasting protective levels. Other vaccines are actually combinations of several unrelated individual vaccines, allowing us to reduce the number of injections a child needs. The combination vaccine we give for diphtheria, tetanus, and whooping cough (the DaPT shot) is an example of this.

Allergies are caused by a division of the immune system that works a little bit differently, although it makes use of antibodies. The particular antibodies involved in allergies (called *immunoglobulin E antibodies*) are not directed against viruses or bacteria. Instead they bind to things from the environment called *allergens*, examples of which include ragweed and goldenrod pollen, insect venom such as from bees, and food products such as nuts or shellfish.

The first time or two a child's body encounters an allergen, not much happens. Over time, however, the antibodies to the allergen coat the surfaces of specialized cells called *mast cells*. These cells are concentrated in certain tissues—the skin, the lining of the nose, and the respiratory passages are particularly rich in them. Not surprisingly, these are places where allergic symptoms commonly happen. Many of the mast cells in a person allergic to ragweed, for example, are covered with an immunoglobulin E antibody that recognizes ragweed.

A good way to think of a mast cell is as an alert guard who doggedly waits for a very specific target. And this particular guard is armed with a lot of weapons. These are contained within packets inside the cell. When the mast cell feels its particular enemy touch the antibody tripwires on its surface, something we call *activation*, it launches its entire arsenal. The substances in this arsenal cause all the symptoms we experience as allergies.

Foremost among the things an activated mast cell lets loose into its surrounding tissue is a molecule called *histamine*. You read a bit about that substance in chapter 10 about rashes because histamine causes hives. Mast cells tend to congregate around small blood vessels. When they release histamine, it causes a large increase in the diameter of nearby blood vessels, resulting in engorgement of the vessels with blood. Histamine also creates holes, gaps between the cells lining the vessels. Together, this causes immediate swelling and redness in the surrounding tissues. In the skin, mast cells also gather near nerve endings, where released histamine causes the nerve stimulation we know as itching.

Histamine is an incredibly powerful substance. If large amounts of it get into the bloodstream it can cause a catastrophe because it can do to the entire body what is does locally in an allergic response. A sudden increase in blood-vessel diameter throughout the body does the same thing to a person's blood pressure that suddenly quadrupling the diameter of the cold water pipes in your house would do to your household water pressure: a fixed amount of fluid now needs to occupy a significantly larger space, so there is less fluid pressure. If you had your shower running, you would notice an immediate drop in water flow. When histamine does a similar thing to the body's blood vessels, making them larger, the overall blood pressure can fall dramatically. Such a major drop in blood pressure can have profound effects on the body, some of them potentially serious.

Histamine from the mast cells that normally live in the breathing passages can have serious effects too. It can bring on swelling of the tongue and soft tissues around the back of the throat, blocking airflow. It may cause intense tightening of those tiny muscular nooses around the small airways you read about in chapter 5, leading to an asthma attack. It is this property of histamine that forms the link between allergies and asthma for some people. Although histamine is the main actor in this cellular drama, the mast cells have several other potent substances they release along with it that also cause the tissues to become inflamed.

Serious or even life-threatening allergic reactions are rare, but they can happen. Thankfully, most of the time histamine and the other mast-cell products only act locally, rather than throughout the body. So generally the effects just cause symptoms in the local environment. For the airway, these include sneezing and a runny nose, or hay fever; for the skin, we see red, itchy swellings—hives.

Everybody knows that some people have allergies, others do not. Why is that? The answer is that the immune system in general, and especially the part of it which controls immunoglobulin E and the mast cells, is highly determined by genetics, by the tendencies we inherit from our parents. Many people can breathe in ragweed pollen for years and never make any antibody to it, never prime their mast cells to react to it. But some people do. For those people, the symptoms often get progressively worse over the years because their populations of primed mast cells get higher and higher.

Fortunately for allergy sufferers, we have several effective treatments that improve the situation. We cannot cure the problem, but we usually can control the troublesome symptoms. These treatments attack the problem from several different angles. Some specifically counteract the effects of histamine and the other mast-cell products. Others work more generally to dampen the effects these substances cause. Still others work by reducing the ability of mast cells to become activated in the first place.

Antihistamines are common medicines. They work just as the name implies—they neutralize histamine. The traditional antihistamine for many decades was diphenhydramine (Benadryl, many others). This still works, but it has the side effect of causing drowsiness. More recently researchers have devised antihistamines that cause little or no drowsiness. Two common examples of these are cetirizine (Zyrtec, many others) and loratadine (Claritin, many others).

Another way to control allergies is to use drugs that block tissue inflammation. These drugs do not interfere with histamine directly, but they both inhibit the ability of mast cells to release their contents and block the effects of inflammatory mast-cell components after they are released.

A standard medicine for doing this is called a *corticosteroid*. We can give steroids in several ways. For chronic nasal allergies, we can spray steroids inside the nose, where their effect is only in that area. Given that way, steroids are safe for prolonged use. For more pronounced allergic attacks, such as severe hives, we can give steroids systemically as liquids, pills, or injections. When given in one of those ways, steroids are extremely potent blockers of allergic symptoms, but they also can have unwanted side effects for the body if they are used for more than a few days at a time. They are safe for episodic use, but they are not appropriate as therapy for chronic conditions.

We also have a very potent blocker of allergic symptoms in the form of the hormone *epinephrine*. This hormone is normally made by the adrenal glands, which is why it is also called *adrenaline*. Epinephrine shrinks swollen blood vessels very quickly, so allergic-tissue swelling dramatically improves. However, we reserve epinephrine for serious or emergency situations, and it must be injected through a needle. If your child ever has an allergic reaction that requires a 911 call, this is what the paramedics will treat the problem with. Families with children who have severe allergies, such as to bee stings, often are given a preloaded, auto-injectable syringe of epinephrine to give their child in an emergency (brand names EpiPen and EpiPen Jr).

For children with more severe allergies, there is another treatment mode that can work if the specific allergen is known. It is called *desensitization*. This method works by giving the child a series of injections containing increasingly larger doses of the allergen. When the body sees the allergen in this way, it uses another arm of the immune system, a different class of antibodies than the immunoglobulin E class of allergies, to bind to the allergen. The effect of this is to use the other antibodies to hide the allergen from the mast-cell system. If the mast cells cannot see the allergen, they cannot react to it. If the primed mast cells go through many months or years of not seeing their target allergen, they also reduce their numbers.

Desensitization treatment, however, is complicated. It requires that the specific allergen for a particular child be known. We determine that by skin tests in which minute amounts of the allergen are scratched into the skin to see if there is a little reaction. Once the allergen (or allergens) is identified, it takes many months of regular injections to achieve results, so this treatment is not useful for acute or sudden allergic reactions. For some children, though, desensitization therapy is extremely useful. It is usually administered by specialist physicians called *allergists*.

Parents, and even physicians sometimes, toss around the term *allergy* when what they are describing is really not an allergy. So before we get to specific scenarios, it is worth first talking a little bit about what is not an allergy. A true allergy needs to involve the system you have just read about. There are many things that can make a child uncomfortable, but most of them are not allergies because they do not work by way of the immunoglobulin E and mast-cell system. Now on to the case scenarios to put these principles into action.

WATCHFUL WAITING

Your ten-year-old has spent a windy summer weekend visiting his cousins on your brother's farm. When he returns on Sunday evening he has a rash all over his abdomen, chest, and upper arms. It itches quite a bit, and he has been scratching, causing a few scabs here and there. He also has a stuffy nose, but otherwise has no problems breathing—no cough or shortness of breath. He enjoyed the weekend but seems pretty uncomfortable from these symptoms. Should you bring him to the doctor tonight? Should you wait until morning and see if he still has these symptoms? Is there anything you can do tonight to make him feel better?

What has happened to this child fits very well with a reaction to something he encountered on the farm. Even though he has not had any allergic reactions before, the dose of allergen he encountered over the weekend was probably quite high, and he probably was sensitized in the past from meeting lower doses. There are many possibilities, ranging from plant materials like hay and grass to animal hair and dander.

It really does not matter now which of these was the culprit; if this were your child, there are some things you could do to make him feel better. The first is to wash him and his clothes thoroughly to get rid of residual allergen, whatever it was. You could then give him an over-the-counter antihistamine to block the allergic reaction. Benadryl (and its many generic equivalents) is available both as a liquid and as a capsule. The proper dose is on the box or bottle, but it is around one-half milligram per pound of body weight. You could also apply an anti-inflammatory cream to the itchy rash, something also available without prescription. One percent hydrocortisone cream can be found in any pharmacy and most grocery stores. The bottom line in this scenario is that you definitely could make him feel better without dragging him to the emergency department. If you did, they would most likely recommend the measures you just read about.

CALL THE DOCTOR

Your eight-year-old daughter has had nasal allergies for several years—a chronic runny nose during the late summer and fall. Her doctor has diagnosed her with seasonal plant allergies, since that time of the year is when the pollen count is highest, and she takes cetirizine (Zyrtec) every day during those months. It is August and her symptoms have been a bit worse for the past several days. Tonight she has added a cough to her symptom list. You think she also may be a bit short of breath, although she is not breathing fast. She mainly seems a bit less energetic than usual. What can you do about this? Does she need more allergy medications now? Does her cough mean she needs to see a doctor tonight?

The key to this scenario is to assess the breathing problem. It is possible her allergies have progressed beyond just inflaming her nose to involving her lower airways too. However, if she does not get any worse than this—not short of breath, not breathing fast, not experiencing chest tightness—then it is reasonable to observe how she does for now. If this were your daughter, it would be best to call her doctor for advice and perhaps arrange for an evaluation. She might benefit from an additional oral allergy medication or occasional use of a medication such as albuterol when she has breathing symptoms (you read about albuterol in chapter 5).

GO TO THE EMERGENCY DEPARTMENT

Your four-year-old son has been playing in the backyard all morning. He just ran into the house crying, saying that he was stung by bees. You look at the back of his hand and see it is quite red and swollen from at least one sting. His other forearm is also swollen, and it looks as if several bees stung him there too. That arm is quite swollen from his wrist to his elbow. He continues to cry, but he does not have any trouble breathing. What should you do?

If this were your son, the range of options is broad, going from watchful waiting to calling 911. It all depends upon how severe the symptoms are. The thing to keep in mind with this scenario is if he has any breathing problems or swelling of his lips or tongue. A very useful indicator is his voice. Is it normal, or is it hoarse or changed in any other way? If it is hoarse or changed, this suggests some potentially dangerous airway swelling. In this case, the child has uncomfortable and painful swelling from multiple bee stings, but he has no breathing problems, so it would be reasonable for you to take him to the emergency department yourself.

The doctors in the emergency department will be able to improve his symptoms very quickly with some of the medications you read about earlier. The pain and swelling would ultimately pass on its own, but we can speed things along substantially. Meanwhile, you can help by putting an ice pack on the affected areas. This helps with the pain and swelling by slowing down inflammation.

CALL 911

Your family is eating out in a restaurant. Your nine-year-old son is curious to try lobster. He would like one of the live ones in the tank at the side of the dining room, but the occasion is not *that* special. He settles for a dish containing bits of lobster in a cream sauce. About fifteen minutes after starting the dinner, he says he feels funny; his lips and tongue feel thick. You also notice his voice seems a bit hoarse, and it sounds as if his breathing is becoming labored and difficult. You tell him to stop eating the dinner, since you appropriately suspect he is developing some sort of reaction to it. Other than that, what should you do? Perhaps give him some water to wash the food down and clear his mouth?

If this were your child, the answer to the scenario is you should spoil everyone's dinner by pulling out your cell phone and calling 911. He is most likely developing a severe reaction to his dinner, probably the lobster because shellfish is a common allergy. Most of these reactions are mild. But the particular symptoms he is experiencing suggest he is at risk for developing very severe breathing problems very quickly. He needs attention as soon as possible, and paramedics   carry   medications—especially   epinephrine—to counteract a developing allergic reaction. These medications are very effective, and the odds are overwhelming your son will be fine. After this episode is over, though, and you have gone home from the emergency department, you should take him to the doctor for an evaluation and a discussion about how to prevent this problem in the future.

CHECKLIST AND ACTION PLANS FOR ALLERGIES

The most important principle in this chapter is attention to the severity of the symptoms, especially breathing troubles. You can apply to allergic reactions many of the principles you learned in chapter 5.

Watchful Waiting

1. Your child has a rash but not much swelling.
2. Your child has itching, but it is relatively mild.
3. Your child has no breathing symptoms, no shortness of breath.
4. Your child's symptoms have come on slowly—over hours, not minutes.

Call the Doctor

1. Your child's symptoms are recurrent.
2. Your child has more-severe itching.

Go to the Emergency Department

1. Your child has widespread swelling.
2. Your child has symptoms of breathing problems.

3. Your child has no swelling of the lips or tongue.
4. There is no change in your child's voice.

Call 911

1. Your child has rapid and noticeable swelling of the lips or tongue.
2. Your child's voice is hoarse or raspy.
3. Your child is wheezing and short of breath.

14

OTHER MISCELLANEOUS CONDITIONS

In the previous chapters you read about a wide variety of illnesses and injuries that cause parents to wonder if they should bring their child to the emergency department. They were all grouped logically according to organ systems, such as the lungs and airway, the brain, and the skin. That approach does cover the great majority of situations. However, there are inevitably things we occasionally see in the emergency department that do not easily fit into the categories you have already read about. This chapter is about some of those, although of course the list cannot be exhaustive. The situations do not lend themselves to the sort of checklist-based format we have used in the previous chapters, but I think you will find that reading a scenario about each of them will make it clear what to do should you encounter one of these situations with your child.

SCENARIO 1: A BABY WITH A FAST HEART RATE

This scenario involves a six-week-old infant. He has been well up to now, with a normal birth experience. One morning his mother notices that he is feeding less well than usual. Over the course of the day, as she tries to feed him, she notices he seems to be a little short of breath. This mostly shows itself when he tries to nurse—he breathes faster, forty to fifty breaths per minute, and he can suckle for only a couple of minutes at a time. His mother is concerned, of course, but also perplexed. She knows that most breathing issues in a previously healthy infant are from infections, usually viral, but her baby has not been sick at all. He has had no congestion or runny nose, and no cough.

Then she happens to lay her hand on his chest, and it appears to her that his heart rate is very fast. Worried, she calls her child's doctor, who tells her how to count the heart rate: she can count the beats in fifteen seconds and multiply by four, or count the beats in thirty seconds and double it. This yields the heart rate, which is measured in beats per minute.

The normal heart rate for an infant varies. An agitated baby or one with a fever will have a higher heart rate, but a sustained resting heart rate of over two hundred is abnormal. When the mother counts out the beats, she notes nearly sixty beats in fifteen seconds. That makes a heart rate of about 240. She calls her doctor back with that information, and he tells her to bring the baby to the emergency department. The child still looks fairly well in spite of his fast heart rate, although he continues to breathe faster than normal.

This baby has a not-uncommon problem. It carries the medical name of *supraventricular tachycardia*, or SVT for short. It is a condition in which the electrical system of the heart abruptly develops a short circuit. Normally each heartbeat originates in a specialized part of the upper area of the heart that works as a kind of stopwatch. This part of the heart regularly ticks out electrical impulses that travel down a bundle of tissue wires to a way station in the center of the heart. Think of this way station as an electrical substation. The impulse fans out from the substation over a network of smaller wires that stimulate the heart muscle to beat. Each original signal from the master stopwatch at the top of the heart results in one heartbeat.

In SVT there is a problem in the area of the substation. The electrical impulses passing through and driving heartbeats can establish what we term a *reentry circuit* in which a signal travels backward along aberrant wiring, then enters the main wiring and causes another heartbeat too soon. The result is the abnormally fast heart rate of SVT. The tendency to have this happen is something people are born with, although people who have it can go for many years before having such a spell of increased heart rate.

The problem with the fast heart rate is that it overworks the heart. The heart is a pump. It has four chambers, but it is the two lower, muscular ones (the *ventricles*) that squeeze blood out to the lungs and the rest of the body with each beat. If the heart rate is too fast, the ventricles do not have time to fill completely between beats, which inhibits the normal forward flow of blood. Sometimes blood can back up into the lungs, causing problems with breathing. That is what is starting to happen with this infant.

How to handle this situation is well known, and any emergency department that cares for children will know what to do. The first thing is to attach heart-monitoring leads to the chest of the child. These display the heart rhythm on a screen or print it on paper strips. The pattern of SVT is very easy to identify. Once we know what the problem is, we fix it by resetting the way the substation is processing the electrical impulses. It is not an exact analogy, but you can compare what we do to what you might do if your computer were hung up in an endless loop trying to process something; to fix it, you reboot the computer, allowing it to reload the software. To fix SVT, we reboot the electrical system of the heart.

Often we can use a natural reflex of the nerves that go to the heart by stimulating the ones whose job it is to slow down heart rate. For an infant, the best way to do this is to apply an ice-cold cloth or bag of crushed ice to the infant's face. That triggers the reflex. If that does not work, we have a medicine we inject into a vein that slows heart rate, allowing the normal substation pathway to reestablish itself. If several doses of the medication do not do the trick, which is unusual, we rarely have to apply a brief external electrical shock to the heart. Of course, once the doctors have stopped the SVT episode, the child should be seen by a *cardiologist*, a heart expert. Daily medicine can prevent SVT from happening again. After a time the medicine can often be stopped if the child has no further episodes.

SVT is not rare. In my practice I see several new cases each year. If your small child is looking pale and out of sorts and is perhaps breathing faster than usual, you should check his heart rate. The threshold we generally use as clearly abnormal and requiring medical attention is a rate of two hundred beats per minutes in the absence of things we know boost the heart rate, such as pain, agitation, or fever. If you are in doubt, it is best to call your doctor for advice.

SCENARIO 2: A BABY WHO WILL NOT STOP CRYING

This scenario also concerns a baby. She is two months old and was completely fine until this morning. She is an active baby and waves her arms and legs around a lot. This morning her mother went to pick her up to feed her, and other than being hungry, the infant looked fine. A couple of minutes later, though, she began to cry vigorously—screaming in a way she had never done before. She appeared to her mother to be in considerable pain. Her mother could not discover any clues that would explain the infant's sudden distress. She had been completely alert and herself before. After spending over an hour trying to sooth her infant, the distraught mother called her physician for advice.

The doctor could not explain the baby's symptoms either, but of course that would be difficult to do over the telephone. He told her to continue to observe the child for a few hours, but if the baby did not calm down by then to take her to the emergency department for an evaluation.

Over the next several hours the child would briefly stop crying, but would then soon start again. This child's mother was an experienced one, having had several babies already, and she had never seen any of her other children behave this way before. The child's crying was loud and insistent. She was red in the face and copious tears rolled down from her eyes. One of the child's brothers had had colic as an infant and was quite fussy from that until it passed as he grew older, but his baby sister's degree of distress was much, much more than that. The infant refused her next feeding because of her symptoms, and that was enough for her mother; she took her daughter, crying all the way, to the emergency department.

The doctor in the emergency department looked the baby over and could find nothing obvious to cause such distress. She had no bumps or bruises, no abnormalities in her arms and legs. The baby's abdomen was soft and not swollen or tender, an important thing to note since, as you read in chapter 6, various problems of the intestinal tract can cause considerable pain. But this child had been feeding normally and had had her usual number of stools that day. Also, pain from that cause is generally not constant and unremitting—it worsens and improves over periods of five minutes or so. What could be causing this baby's pain?

The doctor had encountered this situation before, and he did a simple test to confirm his suspicions. He put special, numbing drops in the child's eyes and the child calmed down within minutes. She was red-faced and exhausted after her ordeal, but she clearly felt much better.

Once she had calmed down, the doctor put a different sort of drop in her eye, one that contained a special dye called *fluorescein*. Fluorescein also comes on tiny strips of blotter paper that we can touch to the eye surface and let the child's tears spread them around. If there is any tiny nick or scratch on the surface of the eye the dye will stick to the injured spot. We can then see these spots by shining a special ultraviolet lamp on the eye. The injured areas light up as bright green in color.

This infant had a *corneal abrasion*, a scratch on the eye surface, or *cornea*. The cornea is extremely sensitive. Most of us at one time or another have gotten a piece of grit in our eye and know how uncomfortable that feels until our tears wash the grit off the cornea, after which we have sudden relief. If the cornea has a minute scratch on it, the pain continues.

We can greatly reduce the pain by closing the affected eye and moving our eyeball as little as possible, but a baby cannot figure this out. She just knows that her eye hurts—a lot. What the doctor did was to numb the surface of the eye with drops, giving instant relief. At that point he was pretty sure what the problem was, even if he had not been able to find the scratch with the fluorescein test. But the dye confirmed his diagnosis. Another clue was that the affected eye had excessive tears. Even though the child was crying, the amount of tears pouring out of one eye was unusually profuse.

How did this child get a corneal abrasion anyway? The most likely cause was that she caught the surface of her eye with an edge of her fingernail. Babies often have relatively long nails for their size. This baby was an active, enthusiastic infant who waved her arms around in the air when she was happy. She knew immediately that her eye hurt, but of course she could not tell anyone what the problem was.

How do we treat corneal abrasions? Fortunately, the cells on the surface of the eye reproduce themselves extremely fast. Even by the next day this child's symptoms would be greatly improved. Meanwhile we have numbing eye drops or ointment that will ease the pain and allow this child to feed and sleep normally. Deeper injuries to the eye, ones that go below the surface and are the result of more than a scratch, often need the expertise of an eye specialist, an *ophthalmologist*. Emergency department doctors know how to determine if that is necessary, but simple corneal abrasions heal just fine. There will be no effect on the child's future vision.

SCENARIO 3: ANOTHER INFANT WHO WILL NOT STOP CRYING

This baby is three months old. He was also fine this winter morning when his mother got him up, dressed him, and brought him to his usual daycare center. When his mother picked him up in the late afternoon, however, the daycare person told her that over the course of the afternoon, the child had become progressively more fussy. When his mother put him into his car seat he was inconsolable—crying constantly. She could not figure out what could be bothering him. Like the child in the previous scenario, he had never done anything like this before.

He was still crying when they got home. After another hour or two of this his mother, like the mother in the previous scenario, called the doctor for advice. She got the same answer: if it keeps up, or gets worse, she should bring the child to the emergency department for an evaluation. The child's discomfort did get worse, and the mother brought him in.

The doctor there immediately found the problem by doing something the mother had not thought to do—completely undress the child and look at everything. When the doctor pulled the child's socks off it was obvious that one of his toes was swollen and red. It looked like a sausage compared with the other toes. At the base of his swollen toe there was a deep groove dipping into the skin.

This infant had what we call a *hair tourniquet*. It happens when a hair, or sometimes a thread, becomes twisted around a finger or a toe. Toes are the most common. It is not clear precisely how it starts, but there are often hairs or loose threads on the inside of socks. If one of them snags a toe, the hair can twist around it. Of course a baby may feel that happening, but he cannot just take off his socks and untangle the hair. Once the toe becomes swollen, the hair (or thread) forms an ever-tightening noose around the toe; the progressive tissue swelling contributes to this, tightening the noose. By the time the swelling has reached the point it had in this child, no parent can fix it at home.

Like a corneal abrasion, a hair tourniquet is something every emergency department doctor considers when evaluating an infant who is in significant pain with no obvious reason, no history of any injury. Unlike a corneal abrasion, though, a hair tourniquet on a toe is easy to spot just by pulling off the infant's socks. This mother could have done that, but it being winter, this mother had no reason to do so. If you find yourself in a similar situation, take off all your baby's clothes so you can get a close look at everything.

The way we treat a hair tourniquet is straightforward—we get the hair off. That is not always easy to do, however. Depending upon how deep down the groove is containing the hair, sometimes the doctor can grasp it with a tiny forceps and then snip it with a fine pair of scissors. If the hair is not on dangerously tight, that is, not so tight as to threaten the circulation to the toe, sometimes we can use one of several over-the-counter hair removal products to soften and then dissolve away the hair.

If the doctor cannot snag the hair with a forceps, and particularly if the toe has turned dusky enough to suggest that the deep circulation to the toe is threatened, we can cut the hair. This means that we must also make an incision on the side of the toe to get down to the hair. Before doing that we first numb the toe so the child does not feel the incision, and afterward we close the incision with a few stitches. We do not have to do this very often, but as a last resort it does take care of the problem.

SCENARIO 4: A MOST PERSONAL INJURY

This story is about a six-year-old boy. He has been playing in the backyard all afternoon. After holding off nature for a hour or so, he finally runs into the house to go to the bathroom. Like most boys in this situation, he is in a hurry to get back outside. When he is done urinating he quickly and forcefully zips up his pants. *Ouch*—sudden trouble. He has caught the skin of his penis in the metal zipper. He comes running to his mother, who has a look. The skin is deeply caught in the zipper. She gently tries to pull the zipper down, but he cries out before she has been able to improve things at all. He will not let her try again. What can this mother do? This is an emergency of sorts, but does it require a trip to the emergency department? The boy would be mortified, and the mother would be a little uncomfortable herself.

Zipper injuries like this are actually not uncommon, especially in uncircumcised boys, who can snag their foreskin in the metal zipper. I have seen more than a few during my time in the emergency department. There are several methods we use to solve the problem, things parents can try at home before bringing their son to the doctor.

One trick is to coat the area around the trapped skin with mineral oil or Vaseline, then to gently try to pull the zipper down. For myself I have not found this technique to work, but there are reports in the medical literature of others who say it does work much of the time. It is simple to try.

Another technique, one that has worked for me, is to take the zipper apart. This approach does ruin the zipper, but a pair of pants is a small price to pay in this situation. At the bottom of the zipper there is a metal bar joining the two sides. It actually is a flat loop of metal, not a solid bar. If you can get it off, the zipper will fall apart from the bottom. The technique that has worked for me, and which also has been described by others in medical reports, is to wedge a small screwdriver underneath the part of the bar you can see. Wiggle it back and forth to get some space under it. The bar can then be pulled off with a firm hand and a pair of needle-nose pliers. Alternatively, if you have small wire cutters, you can get it into the space and snip the bar, then twist it off. Once the bar is gone, pull apart the zipper from the bottom up toward the trapped skin.

If you do not have these tools or you are too nervous to try, then the only alternative is to bring your son to the emergency department. This problem is common enough that the doctors there will know how to handle it. Afterward, encourage your son to slow down and be careful next time.

15

A PARENT'S GUIDE TO HOW EMERGENCY DEPARTMENTS WORK

You have read a great deal in the previous chapters about which problems a parent can appropriately observe at home, which are best handled with a call to the doctor for advice, and which need evaluation in an emergency department. If you do bring your child to an emergency department, you may find it a bewildering and even frustrating experience. This is especially the case if you do not understand how these places work, how they differ from a doctor's office or a free-standing walk-in clinic. In our final chapter you will learn some of that useful information. It will allow you to make the best use of the facility to get the care your child needs.

As of 2012 there were nearly five thousand hospitals in America with emergency departments that cared for children. Only about 10 percent of those, however, were in hospitals with the ability to provide advanced pediatric care. About half of those, 250 in all, were found in specialized children's hospitals. That is probably not a significant consideration if your child has an easy, straightforward problem. But if your child has a more complicated or challenging problem and you have access to a children's hospital (most are in large cities), then it makes sense to take your child there for care. This is because the doctors in a dedicated children's facility will be experienced in treating all manner of children's ailments. They also will have ready access to whatever special tests or expert advice your child's case might require.

Children's hospitals do account for a disproportionately large number of emergency department visits by children. Even though only 5 percent of emergency departments who see children are located in dedicated children's hospitals, they cared for nearly 30 percent of all children whose parents brought them to one of America's emergency departments. So it appears parents recognize the difference. On the other hand, nearly a third of children cared for in emergency departments across the country are seen in facilities that do not even have the capacity to care for those children if they are sick enough to require admission to the hospital; if the child needs to come into the hospital, the emergency department has to transfer the child to another facility. If your child is quite sick, it seems best to avoid that situation if possible.

I do not mean to imply that a general hospital cannot give good care to children. For families living in smaller communities, access to a dedicated children's emergency department is limited, and the great majority of general emergency departments do a good job taking care of children with uncomplicated problems. But it is something to consider if you live near a children's hospital and have a choice in where to go. You can find where children's hospitals are by looking at the list of the National Association of Children's Hospitals and Related Institutions (www.childrenshospitals.net).

By their very nature, emergency departments are very inefficient and expensive places to deliver care. This is true for patients of all ages. As we have seen, this is because they need to be ready at all times to handle critically ill or injured patients, even if those categories of patients do not appear very often. Emergency departments always must be prepared for worst-case scenarios. This requires the immediate availability of specialized equipment and a host of staff trained and experienced in using it. The staff must have quick access to expensive x-ray and laboratory equipment that is maintained and ready to use around the clock. These considerations mean that all emergency departments have a very high fixed cost, an expense that is independent of the number of patients they are seeing at any given time.

Many facilities have tried to deal with this situation by having a separate walk-in or ambulatory clinic affiliated with the emergency department. Often these clinics are open evenings and weekends, when doctors' offices are generally closed. The idea is to find a middle ground between the sophisticated and expensive capabilities of the emergency department and the more simple environment of a physician's office. If a child who is quite ill comes to a walk-in clinic, the emergency department is nearby to take over the case. The concept makes sense. For some of the scenarios you have read about in this book, the advice "Go to the Emergency Department" could also apply to one of these facilities.

If you take your child to the emergency department, what can you expect to happen? They can be confusing or even chaotic places. Even the waiting rooms, where you can expect to spend quite a bit of time unless you are lucky, are often complicated. There is something else to consider—the high potential for miscommunication. These are often high-volume places, where there is considerable emphasis on through-put, on getting the children seen, treated, and back out the door. When a harried doctor meets parents who have been waiting a long time, often hours, just to get in to see the doctor, both may already be cranky before the interview even starts.

Once you are through the emergency department door and registered with a clerk, the first medical person you and your child will meet is a nurse. The waiting patients are typically sorted by how sick they appear to the nursing staff. It is not first-come-first-served; the sickest get seen first. This is called *triage*, a term derived from a French word meaning to prioritize patients into thirds: the critically ill, the seriously ill, and the not-so-ill. This is how it should be.

The triage nurse typically has only a few minutes, sometimes even less than a minute, to spend with the patient. The nurse will ask you a few questions, glance at your child, and make a quick assessment of how ill your child looks. The nurse will also pay attention to the things you say, no matter how your child looks. For example, if you tell the nurse your child has been vomiting blood, that will likely move you up on the list.

Sometimes at this point the nurse will check your child's temperature, pulse rate, and breathing rate; sometimes this happens later. If your child is in one of the more-serious tiers of the triage pyramid, the nurse will hustle him to the examination area. If, however, like most children, your child is in the not-so-ill third of the triage pyramid, you will wait to be seen, these days sometimes a very long time.

When you and your child are called back to the examining room, a nurse will again ask you a few questions. You and your child will then wait some more. Since the typical emergency department has many more examining rooms than it has doctors, families wait in one of these rooms until the doctor gets to them. Finally the doctor will come to the examining room door, look at the brief note written by the nurse—which consists of statements like "fever for three days," "coughing for a week," or "vomiting since yesterday"—and then whisk into the room.

You should realize this doctor you are meeting nearly always has other things on her mind besides your child. The doctor in a busy emergency department is typically juggling the problems of several other patients or children in other rooms at the same time she is evaluating your child. For example, she may be thinking about one child sent off to the radiology department for x-rays, about another with blood-test results pending, and perhaps a third awaiting evaluation by a surgeon about possible appendicitis. It is a difficult thing for an emergency department doctor to approach your child with a mind totally cleared of other things—there are built-in competing issues. In a very busy emergency department, it is often nearly impossible to have even a brief interview with a doctor that is not interrupted by others calling the doctor—who for the moment is *your child ' s* doctor—away to the telephone or out into the corridor for some discussion or other.

It is not an ideal system, but it is what we have. It usually works, but it is easy to see how this built-in pressure and chaos can some-times lead to problems.

After the doctor has spoken with you and examined your child, she may be able at that point to figure out what is wrong and decide what to do—give you a prescription for an antibiotic for an ear infection, for example. If the doctor needs tests to determine what to do, that means, depending upon the circumstances, a technician might take a blood sample, a nurse could obtain a urine sample, or you and your child might be sent to the radiology department for x-rays. Generally you and your child will then wait in the examining room for the results to come back. If things are crowded and the examination room is needed for another patient, you might be asked to go back out to the main waiting room.

One of the key reasons for the inefficiency of getting medical care in the emergency department rather than from your usual phy-sician is that the emergency department doctor does not know you and your child. You are strangers to each other. You are also meet-ing each other in a stressful, typically busy place, one where there rarely is time for leisurely conversation. A situation like this is hard-wired for doctors getting more tests than your regular physi-cian might order. This is the one and only time the emergency doctor is going to see you and your child, so the understandable tendency is to get more tests to look for more-serious problems, even if the doctor thinks they are very unlikely.

Another consideration is that most of the time, what the emergency department doctor knows about your child is what you tell her. Medical delivery systems are becoming more and more integrated, especially as electronic medical records become more common, but it is unusual for the doctor to have immediate access to your child's complete past medical record. If she does have such access, and this is something many are striving for, emergency department care instantly becomes more organized and integrated with your child's total health picture. But we have a long way to go before we get to that goal.

If you take your child to an emergency department, what sort of doctor will you meet? As all parents know, a doctor is not a doctor is not a doctor; that is, we are not interchangeable in what we know and what we can do. For most children their regular doctor, if they have one, is either a family doctor or a pediatrician. Some emergency departments, especially those connected to children's hospitals, will have pediatricians in their emergency departments. They often even have highly-trained pediatricians who are experts in the specific specialty of emergency pediatrics. Many smaller emergency departments, especially those found in the communities across rural America, are staffed by family physicians. The doctors in the majority of emergency departments, however, are trained in a relatively new specialty known as *emergency medicine*. What is that, and what might it mean for your child? To answer this important question, you need to know something about how we train physicians.

An aspiring physician, after graduating from college, first goes to medical school, a process that takes four years to complete. There are currently 141 medical schools in the United States, along with 29 osteopathic schools. There were once key distinctions between those categories, but these days they teach essentially the same curriculum and their graduates are eligible for the same specialty training afterward.

The new medical (or osteopathic) graduate is not ready to practice medicine; he must first complete what is known as *residency*. This is a period of anywhere from three to six years or more, depending upon the specialty, during which he is given increasing responsibility to manage patients on his own. At the end of that training, he takes an examination. If he passes, he is then called board-certified in that specialty. Pediatricians complete a three-year residency exclusively devoted to the care of children. Family medicine doctors do a three-year residency that is more broad-based because they expect to care for patients of all ages. The strictly pediatric portion of their training is generally around six months or so. Their pediatric experience necessarily concentrates on common problems in children.

Pediatrics is a very old medical specialty, dating back to the 1920s. Family practice, once called *general practice*, has also been around for a long time. As emergency departments grew in size and complexity, there emerged a brand-new medical specialty to staff them—emergency medicine. Like family doctors, emergency medicine physicians are trained to take care of patients of all ages. However, the focus of their skills is on the problems that bring people to the emergency department. They spend a great deal of their training time learning how to manage potentially life-threatening conditions.

The great majority of people who seek care in an emergency department—85 percent or so—do not have such a problem. They have something that they feel cannot wait, but it is not life-threatening, although they may not know this. Emergency department doctors are experienced in handling a wide variety of acute problems, including problems children have. But the way these physicians are trained inevitably means they will not be the best at dealing with every ailment your child might develop because that is not their focus. They do a good job managing many of the serious things you have read about in this book, but they are not pediatric specialists.

For a parent, this means that if your child has a complicated and specifically pediatric problem that is not a true emergency, unless you are in a dedicated pediatric facility, you will not be seeing a pediatric expert in the emergency department. Most of the time that does not matter much, but sometimes it does. It is certainly something for you to consider when you are deciding whether or not to make a late-night trip to the emergency department.

There is another kind of healthcare provider that a parent may often meet in the emergency department—what we call a *midlevel provider*. Over the past decades our medical delivery system has included people who are not physicians. There are two main categories of these: *nurse practitioners* and *physician assistants*. Both evolved out of the recognition that we have a shortage of primary care physicians. Experts differ over the question of whether or not we actually have a physician shortage in America. Many believe the real issue to be not that we do not have enough physicians, but that we have a poor distribution of doctors—too many subspecialists and not enough primary care doctors like family doctors, pediatricians, and internal medicine practitioners. Whatever the politics of the matter, physician assistants and nurse practitioners emerged to fill this gap. They function in similar roles, but they are not trained in the same way.

A physician assistant is someone who has gone through a specific training program aimed at teaching her how to help physicians by learning to care for patients, including children, with common conditions. The first training programs used former military medics, building upon what they had already learned in the service. A physician assistant has completed a two-to-three-year training program, usually following a college degree. What a graduate of such a program can do varies from state to state. In some places, a physician assistant can function independently of a physician; in other places, physician supervision is required.

A nurse practitioner is somewhat different. These individuals are already trained and certified as nurses. After nursing school they receive several years of additional training to allow them to act in an expanded role beyond nursing. For children, there is a special category called *pediatric nurse practitioner*, or PNP. Such an individual cares only for children. PNPs are widely used in office pediatric practices. Although they usually have some oversight by physicians, their particular skills often allow them to function in a very independent role when taking care of children.

Many emergency departments employ physician assistants, nurse practitioners, or both. Although some physicians continue to have reservations about this arrangement, it makes sense because many of the people seeking care in the emergency department have straightforward, uncomplicated problems that do not require sophisticated medical knowledge to diagnose and treat. A fishhook stuck in a finger, a cut in a hand, or uncomplicated wheezing are examples of these. But parents should know that if they take their child to the emergency department, they may not necessarily see a doctor. As I noted earlier, sometimes that does not matter, but sometimes it does.

What does all of this mean if you decide to take your child to the emergency department? You will be meeting a healthcare provider who does not know your child. He typically will not have any access to previous medical records that will help him know what has happened to your child in the past. All he will know about your child is what you can tell him. So you should think hard about how best to do that. The odds are you will spend some time in the waiting room, which is a good opportunity to organize your thoughts.

Conversation has been the cornerstone of medical care since the time of Hippocrates, the founder of Western medicine over two thousand years ago. For much of that time, talking and listening to patients was in fact *all* the doctor did; the idea that a physician should actually examine a sick patient is an innovation barely a hundred years old. This notion of talking with but never examining a patient appears ridiculous to us, but actually it is based on a great truth—in most cases, doctors decide on what is probably wrong with a patient and what to do about it based upon nothing more than a conversation with the patient. Of course this conversation is more important in some cases than in others. After all, a broken leg is still a broken leg, no matter the circumstances of how it happened. The majority of the time, however, the conversation between physician and patient is where everything starts.

The most useful way you can prepare for the doctor to see your child is to get clear in your own mind the details of your child's problem. It is a good idea to write things down: When did the problem start? Did it change over time? Did you do anything about it, and did that help? Has your child had a similar problem before, and how did that go? The doctor you see is likely busy and will very much appreciate your effort to sort things out. It will also allow him to give your child the best care.

There are several key expectations you should have during your trip to the emergency department. Foremost among these is that you should always understand what is going on. Insist that the doctor explain, in ways you can understand, what the problem is, what needs to be done about it, and what to expect later. Make sure you know what is being done and why. Make sure you know if further doctor visits will be needed afterward. If possible, ask the emergency department to send to your regular doctor a record of what happened there. Many emergency departments do this routinely, but it is always good to ask.

The goal of this book has been to give you, the parent, a working knowledge of how doctors evaluate many common acute problems in children, how we decide things. It is not difficult for any parent to develop some ability to do this, even if the specifics require medical training. Of course this book is not intended to replace medical evaluation, and you should not be practicing medicine on your children. Still, most parents can understand some key principles that will help them decide what to do if their child is sick in the middle of the night.

Good luck, and realize that children are amazingly resilient creatures. They heal very well and grow up to have children of their own.

SUGGESTIONS FOR FINDING FURTHER INFORMATION

GENERAL INFORMATION

These days the most useful sources for further information are online. However, as the saying goes, the Internet is miles wide but inches deep. There is a lot of information out there, but some of it is wrong or inadequate. I have looked at all of the sites I list here, and their information is reliable. There are many useful places to find good advice about children's health. The best ones are maintained by prominent children's hospitals and medical organizations—check at your local children's hospital to see if they have one—but here are some good places to go.

The American Academy of Pediatrics: www.healthychildren.org
The American Academy of Family Physicians: www.aafp.org
The Mayo Clinic: www.mayoclinic.com
Boston Children's Hospital: www.childrenshospital.org
The Children's Hospital of Philadelphia: www.chop.edu
Cincinnati Children's Hospital: www.cincinnatichildrens.org/patients/child/health/
The Children's Hospital of Colorado: www.childrenscolorado.org
Children's Hospital of Los Angeles: www.chla.org
Seattle Children's Hospital: www.seattlechildrens.org
Nemours Children's Hospital: http://kidshealth.org

There are also excellent blogs maintained by pediatricians where you can find reliable information and interact with the blog owner, read about other parents' experiences, and even contribute yourself. This is a rapidly changing area, of course, but here is a sampling of some excellent pediatric blogs that have been around for several years at least and are maintained by pediatricians who frequently post informative essays. None of them pitch products—just simple information exchange.

Dr. Wendy Sue Swanson's blog: http://seattlemamadoc.seattlechildrens.org
Dr. Claire McCarthy's blog: http://childrenshospitalblog.org
Dr. Natasha Burgert's blog: http://kckidsdoc.com
My own blog: www.chrisjohnsonmd.com/blog/

CHAPTER 3: FEVER

The important thing about fever is to understand what it is—a sign of something else and not a disease in itself. Respect it, but do not have "fever phobia." Here are some places where you can find further information.

http://pediatrics.aappublications.org/content/127/3/580.full
www.kevinmd.com/blog/2011/08/fever-children-5-facts.html
www.parenting.com/category/conditions/fever
www.fda.gov/ForConsumers/ConsumerUpdates/ucm263989.htm
www.uptodate.com/contents/fever-in-children-beyond-the-basics

CHAPTER 4: COUGHS, SNEEZES, SORE THROATS, AND EARACHES

Remember that very few of these conditions need immediate treatment in the emergency department. Most do not need any specific treatment at all. Here are some places you can find out more about these common conditions.

http://kidshealth.org/parent/general/eyes/childs_cough.html
http://kidshealth.org/kid/talk/qa/sneeze.html
www.uptodate.com/contents/sore-throat-in-children-beyond-the-basics
www.seattlechildrens.org/medical-conditions/symptom-index/sore-throat/
www.healthychildren.org/English/health-issues/conditions/ear-nose-throat/
    pages/Earaches-and-Your-Child.aspx
www.nidcd.nih.gov/health/hearing/pages/earinfections.aspx

CHAPTER 5: BREATHING TROUBLES

Unlike URI symptoms, breathing troubles in the middle of the night not uncommonly need prompt evaluation. What parents need is guidance in deciding if this is the case with their child. These links will help you do that (some are to my own blog) as well as teach you much more about asthma, croup, pneumonia, and bronchiolitis.

www.uptodate.com/contents/asthma-treatment-in-children-beyond-the-basics
www.chrisjohnsonmd.com/2013/02/08/all-about-croup/
www.chrisjohnsonmd.com/2011/11/08/its-time-once-again-for-bronchiolitis-
    and-respiratory-syncytial-virus-rsv/
http://kidshealth.org/parent/infections/lung/pneumonia.html

CHAPTER 6: DIGESTIVE AND ABDOMINAL PROBLEMS

Most stomach aches and mild-to-moderate diarrhea episodes can be watched at home, but a few need a middle-of-the-night trip to the emergency department. These links will give you more information about the possibility of your child having significant dehydration or other issues that need prompt attention, including the potential for requiring surgery.

http://children.webmd.com/tc/abdominal-pain-age-11-and-younger-topic-over-
    view
www.nlm.nih.gov/medlineplus/ency/article/002466.htm

www.mayoclinic.com/health/dehydration
http://kidshealth.org/parent/firstaid_safe/emergencies/dehydration.html
www.healthychildren.org/English/health-issues/conditions/abdominal/pages/Appendicitis.aspx
www.healthychildren.org/English/health-issues/conditions/abdominal/pages/Abdominal-Pain-in-Children.aspx

CHAPTER 7: BUMPS AND CONKS ON THE HEAD

Additional background information about head injuries is helpful, and a couple of these links contain that. But what a parent really needs help with is deciding if a particular head injury is worrisome enough that they should take their child to the emergency department. Several of these links will help you do that.

http://kidshealth.org/parent/firstaid_safe/emergencies/head_injury.html#
www.uptodate.com/contents/head-injury-in-children-and-adolescents-beyond-the-basics
www.childrenshospital.org/az/Site985/mainpageS985P0.html
www.healthychildren.org/English/health-issues/injuries-emergencies/pages/Head-Injury.aspx

CHAPTER 8: SPRAINS, DISLOCATIONS, AND BROKEN BONES

Most of these injuries are minor and do not need an emergency department visit. Even those injuries that need attention can often wait until morning. But for some children, the emergency department can provide treatment that makes them feel better quicker. For a few children, such as those with broken bones, a prompt trip to the emergency department is necessary. These links will help you decide which of those categories describes your child.

www.chop.edu/healthinfo/sprains-and-strains.html
www.chw.org/display/PPF/DocID/22592/router.asp
http://orthoinfo.aaos.org/topic.cfm?topic=a00039

http://orthoinfo.aaos.org/topic.cfm?topic=A00424
http://reference.medscape.com/features/slideshow/pediatric-fractures
http://kidshealth.org/parent/general/aches/b_bone.html
www.cincinnatichildrens.org/health/f/fractures/

CHAPTER 9: CUTS, LACERATIONS, AND OTHER SKIN INJURIES

As you read in chapter 9, any but the most superficial lacerations are best taken care of in the emergency department soon after they happen. Simple burns can often be managed at home, but some of them also need prompt attention. These links give you more detailed information about what to do for your child. The last link in the list is a video of how lacerations are repaired.

www.chop.edu/healthinfo/lacerations-with-stitches.html
www.childrenshospital.org/az/Site1216/mainpageS1216P0.html
www.aafp.org/afp/2008/1015/p945.html
www.safedragon.com/htmlfold/contents/emergen/experts/emergenexpert.html
www.youtube.com/watch?v=r3sLn6Zu9H8

CHAPTER 10: RASHES

Very few rashes need a trip to the emergency department. Chapter 10 described categories of rashes, but pictures are the best description. These links all have them. The last link gives you a picture of petechiae, the serious rash that does need a doctor's prompt evaluation.

www.emedicinehealth.com/skin_rashes_in_children/article_em.htm
http://children.webmd.com/ss/slideshow-common-childhood-skin-problems
www.seattlechildrens.org/kids-health/page.aspx?id=60253
http://children.webmd.com/tc/rash-age-11-and-younger-topic-overview
www.mayoclinic.com/health/petechiae/MY01104

CHAPTER 11: OVERDOSES, POISONINGS, AND BITES

As you learned in this chapter, the most important thing to know about overdoses and poisonings, and serious bites too, is the number of Poison Control. Once again, that number is 1-800-222-1222. There are a vast number of things children can ingest. These links give you more information about many of the common ones. The last link on the list is about venomous-snake bites.

www.aafp.org/afp/2009/0301/p397.html
www.medscape.com/viewarticle/589474
www.mayoclinic.com/health/acetaminophen/ho00002/nsectiongroup=2
www.hopkinsmedicine.org/healthlibrary/conditions/pediatrics/
   snake_bites_and_children_90,P02849/

CHAPTER 12: HEADACHES, CONVULSIONS, AND ALTERED MENTAL STATES

Headaches are common and rarely need immediate attention, but convulsions, or seizures, are not so common and generally do need a doctor's prompt evaluation. Persistent alteration in a child's level of awareness also generally needs prompt attention. These links give more information about how a child's brain works and what to do if your child develops problems with his. The last link is about ALTEs.

www.mayoclinic.com/health/headaches-in-children/DS01132
www.childrenshospital.org/az/Site986/mainpageS986P0.html
www.epilepsyfoundation.org/livingwithepilepsy/parentsandcaregivers/parents/
   typesofseizures.cfm
http://pediatrics.uchicago.edu/chiefs/inpatient/ALTE.htm

CHAPTER 13: ALLERGIC REACTIONS

Some severe allergic reactions require a visit to the emergency department, or even a 911 call. These links tell you more about allergies, including additional background about what they are and what we do to treat them.

www.chw.org/display/PPF/DocID/21539/router.asp
http://kidshealth.org/parent/firstaid_safe/emergencies/anaphylaxis.html
http://kidshealth.org/parent/medical/allergies/allergy.html
www.childrenshospital.org/az/Site924/mainpageS924P0.html
www.ncbi.nlm.nih.gov/pubmedhealth/PMH0001815/

INDEX

ABOUT THE AUTHOR

Christopher M. Johnson, MD, is a physician trained in pediatrics, infectious diseases, hematology research, and pediatric critical care medicine. He has over thirty years of experience caring for children in the emergency department and the pediatric intensive care unit. He is a former professor of pediatrics at Mayo Medical School and director of Pediatric Critical Care Medicine at the Mayo Clinic. He is the author of more than a hundred medical research papers, as well as three other medical books for general readers: *Your Critically Ill Child: Life and Death Choices Parents Must Face*; *How to Talk to Your Child's Doctor: A Handbook for Parents*; and *How Your Child Heals: An Inside Look at Common Childhood Ailments*.